PSYCHIATRY
made ridiculously simple

by
Jefferson E Nelson, MD
Distinguished Life Fellow of the
American Psychiatric Association
Austin, Texas

William V Good, MD
Senior Scientist
Smith-Kettlewell Eye Research Institute
San Francisco, California

Michael Ascher, MD
Clinical Assistant Professor
Perelman School of Medicine at the
University of Pennsylvania
Philadelphia, Pennsylvania

Art by Don P Bridge, DDS

MedMaster, Inc., Miami

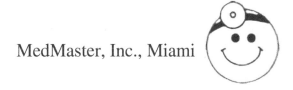

ISBN # 978-1-935660-13-2

Made in the United States of America

Published by
MedMaster, Inc.
P.O. Box 640028
Miami, FL 33164

DEDICATION

*To Phyllis, Alex, Jack, Laurie, Benjamin,
Samuel, Lauren, and Jordana*

CONTENTS

Preface to the 5th Edition vii

1. Introduction. 1

2. Psychiatric Evaluation. 6

3. The Depressed and Suicidal Patient 11

4. Psychoses 21

5. Bipolar Disorder. 28

6. Delirium/Dementia. 33

7. The Anxious Patient 36

8. Alcohol and Substance Use Disorders 44

9. The Sleepless Patient. 52

10. Eating Disorders. 57

11. Pain 63

12. Medical Problems Presenting as Psychiatric Syndromes 68

13. Psychiatric Conditions of Childhood 74

14. The Patient with Sexual Problems 83

15. Personality Disorders 87

16. Treatment Modalities 92

17. Clinical Review 116

Appendix: Suggested Readings 128

Index 129

PREFACE TO THE 5th EDITION

We hope that this book will be a useful manual for students and practitioners from all disciplines (including medicine, nursing, psychology, social work, and occupational therapy). Our aim is to help readers grasp the fundamentals of psychiatry and facilitate retention of key concepts. For those interested in a more extensive understanding of a particular topic, please keep an eye out for suggested additional readings.

Developing an understanding of the psychological jargon is necessary for communicating effectively with mental health professionals. Throughout the book we will be highlighting some of the common terms in psychiatry, including the DSM-5 (Diagnostic and Statistical Manual of Mental Disorders, Fifth Edition, American Psychiatric Association, 2013)

CHAPTER 1.   INTRODUCTION

Psychiatry focuses on the evaluation and treatment of mental disorders, and it intersects many areas of medicine and social sciences including neurology, psychology, neuroscience, public health, and cultural anthropology to name a few. Formal psychiatric specialities include child and adolescent, forensic, addiction, geriatric, and consultation-liaison. Psychiatrists can also choose to practice in many different settings and areas such as community psychiatry, cultural psychiatry, sports psychiatry, neurobehavioral psychiatry, family psychiatry, women's mental health, bioethics, and neurobiological research, depending on their particular interests and strengths. The ability to work in an interdisciplinary setting with psychologists, nurse practitioners, social workers, occupational therapists, and other physicians is a necessary skill in the modern practice of psychiatry.

Recent advances in neuroscience have put to rest the outdated notions of mind-body duality. Memory and learning are the result of neurochemical changes in the brain. Years ago, popular opinion assumed that psychiatrists mainly dealt with sex, a la Sigmund Freud; more recently this view was that psychiatrists only prescribe drugs. In fact, everything we do affects the nervous system. So whether the treatment is a drug, psychotherapy sessions, or directed activity, the brain is changed in the process.

Psychiatric training emphasizes, first and foremost, the establishment of a therapeutic relationship with the patient based on trust, empathy and respect.

The 5th Edition DSM

The 5th edition of the *Diagnostic and Statistical Manual of Mental Disorders* (DSM-5) of the American Psychiatric Association (APA) was released in May 2013, but it remains a work in progress, designed at the outset to undergo continuous revision. The hope is that the DSM-5 will more clearly inform treatment planning, medication choices, protocols, insurance reimbursements, and research agendas. The DSM-5 now highlights both the presence of symptoms and their severity. It is also worth noting that the change away from the traditional Roman numerals of previous editions was intentional. According to the DSM-5 website, this "...change reflects APA's intention to make future revision processes more responsive to breakthroughs.... incremental updates will be identified with decimals, i.e., DSM-5.1, DSM-5.2, etc., until a new edition is required."

The Bio-Psychosocial Model

A bio-psychosocial model is used to explain and describe the development of psychiatric disorders. This theory takes into consideration the individual's physical and genetic endowment, his or her psychological development, and cultural and/or social factors in the manifestation of the illness. The interplay of all 3 over time accounts for the development of psychiatric disorders.

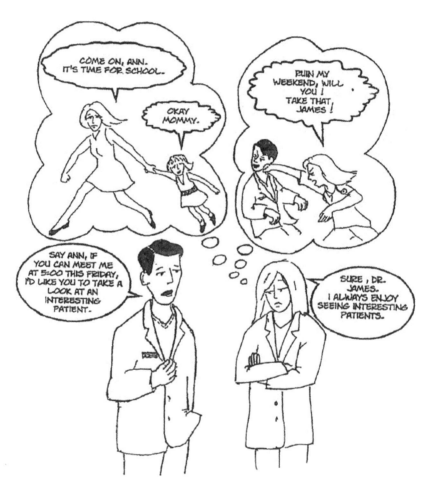

Fig. 1-1. Conflict between wanting to slug the resident and holding back; transference of mother-child and resident-student roles.

We'll try to illustrate some of these factors with the example of a third-year medical student who is feeling particularly depressed late on a Friday afternoon because she had been hoping to go out with friends that night. The situation is that her resident has just suggested that they go to see an interesting new patient who has just been admitted to the ICU. The psychological issues here may be approached from a *psychodynamic perspective* or a *cognitive therapy perspective*. Cognitive therapy is based on the cognitive model, i.e., thoughts and beliefs influence feelings, which influence behaviors. In the more biochemical view, the consideration of neurotransmitters and brain regions comes into focus. Psychodynamically the medical student struggles with the internal conflict of anger at the resident versus that anger turned toward herself, leading to depressed mood and psychological defenses such as reaction formation or identification with the aggressor (see Chapter 16 for further descriptions of defenses).

Viewed from the cognitive model, the medical student thinks, "I'm not worth having a real (social) life anyway, all I'm good for is to do his dirty work," and she trudges off following the resident.

Neurophysiologically, the medical student may be suffering from more severe depressive symptoms that imply dysfunction in neurotransmitter pathways.

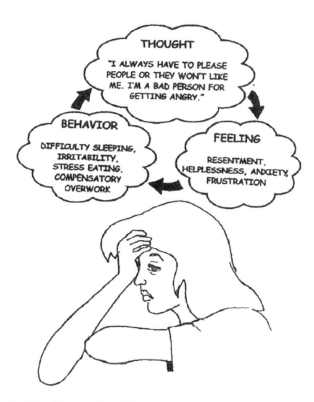

Fig. 1-2. The cognitive triad.

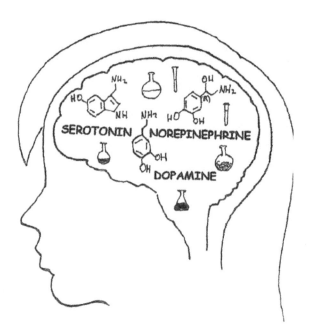

Fig. 1-3.   Serotonin, norepinephrine, and dopamine.

Professionalism and Confidentiality

Psychiatrists are asked to manage a variety of different kinds of patients in a variety of different settings. Working in the hospital with patients and staff may be especially challenging. Psychiatrists are often called to medical and surgical units to make treatment recommendations that may include a patient's capacity to make life-and-death decisions, such as refusing medical interventions. To have the capacity to refuse or accept a medical intervention, the patient must be able to comprehend and communicate an understanding of the risks, benefits, and alternatives to the proposed treatment.

Although psychiatrists are geared to manage mental illness, they are also called upon to help negotiate other difficult situations that may arise in busy medical or hospital practices. Disagreements between nursing staff, physicians, or administrative personnel can be a part of the psychiatrist's domain. Unfortunately, sometimes psychiatrists are asked to function as sanitation engineers in the hospital. "Get this patient off my back" is an occasional request made by a referring physician to a psychiatrist. "This patient wants to sue me—make him stop feeling that way" is a psychiatrist-as-brainwasher view of the specialty.

Generally, a psychiatrist should become involved in a psychologically difficult or psychologically related case early on in management. Early psychiatric intervention helps prevent the patient from feeling that he has been "dumped" by his regular physician and elevates psychiatric illness to a respectable position in the

4

patient's mind. This requires that psychiatric illness have a respectable position in the primary physician's mind!

As clinicians, we are in a powerful role, and our patients put significant trust in us to embrace the ethical principles of *non-malfeasance (do no harm)* and *beneficence (to heal)*. Another important ethical principle is *fidelity*, which means that it's the clinician's duty to place the patient's welfare above all else. While it is important to be nice, caring, and helpful, we must also act in a way that is beneficial to the patient in the long term. In most clinical situations we must try to avoid patients becoming too reliant on us and model ways of relating that stress the importance of having a healthy separation between the self and others. In order to avoid the clinical, legal, and ethical problems that may occur when personal boundaries are crossed or violated, we must continually take a step back and think about whether a certain action is in the best interests of the patient.

No introduction to the field of psychiatry would be complete without a discussion about *confidentiality*. It's striking how many physicians disregard this important concept. Suffice it to say that the topic of conversation in a psychiatrist's office is usually not the local weather forecast. The physician, privy to important and potentially embarrassing information concerning his patient, must do everything possible to safeguard his patient's privacy and his relationship with the patient. Otherwise, the patient will lose trust in his doctor, and all hope of getting to the root of his problems will be gone. There are only two circumstances in which a clinician may breach confidentiality: 1) When a court orders the clinician to testify, to be deposed, or to produce a patient's medical chart; or 2) When a patient poses a threat to himself or herself or to another identifiable individual. However, confidentiality is both an ethical and a legal responsibility. Several federal laws, including HIPAA, direct healthcare professionals concerning confidentiality. State laws also govern the parameters of disclosure of confidential information, and practitioners must learn how to comply with the applicable requirements in the jurisdiction where they work.

CHAPTER 2. PSYCHIATRIC EVALUATION

As in all of medicine, the initial evaluation of the patient is critical to proper diagnosis and effective treatment. In psychiatry, whether you are seeing a quietly depressed patient in the office or an agitated and angry person in the emergency room, the engagement of the patient in a nonjudgmental and open manner (being mindful of your tone of voice, body language, and eye contact) is essential to eliciting a complete history of the presenting problems and details of the past history.

The psychiatrist must evaluate the patient's *symptoms* (subjective experiences reported by the patient, e.g., pain, hearing voices) and *signs* (objective manifestations observed by clinicians) and gather historical information from a biopsychosocial perspective to adequately evaluate the patient. The onset of symptoms, precipitating and ameliorating factors, and the context in which they appear are critical pieces of information to elicit. The patient's personal and family history of illnesses as well as life traumas are particularly relevant. The development of a differential diagnosis depends on an understanding of the key features of psychiatric diagnoses that are currently detailed in DSM-5. The initial diagnostic impression will lead to a treatment plan addressing the need for psychotropic medication (bio), psychotherapy (psycho), and social interventions (social).

Format for Psychiatric Evaluations

Patient Identification:
Chief Complaint:
History of Present Illness:
Past Psychiatric History: treatment, including medications and hospitalization; past suicidal or homicidal behavior; family psychiatric history; substance use history
Past Medical History and Surgical History:
Current Home Meds/Supplements/Vitamins:
Allergies (Type):
Social: childhood; education; marital; occupational; legal
Physical Exam: (if available)

Mental Status Exam (MSE): (see below)
  A: *Appearance/affect* and mood
  B: *Behavior*
  S: *Speech*
  T: *Thought process*
  R: *Reasoning* and judgment
  A: *Attention* and memory
  C: *Cognition*, including orientation and intellectual functioning
  T: *Thought content*

A crucial part of our examination is the mental status exam, which substitutes for the physical exam. Ideally the patient will have had a history and physical exam and appropriate laboratory tests by his or her primary care physician.

As a rule of thumb, the mental status examination and other questions that cover cognition, attention, and memory should not be performed at the beginning of an interview with the patient unless the patient is grossly disoriented (unable to describe the current time and place). Some effort should be made to converse and develop an alliance with the patient prior to asking questions that may make the patient feel embarrassed.

Certain fundamental questions should be asked and observations made concerning every patient you evaluate. The mnemonic, **ABSTRACT**, is provided to help organize your thinking, and we've included a review of quick and simple ways for testing various parts of the mental status examination. Remember, this mental status exam is a snapshot of the patient at a particular moment.

A: *Appearance/affect and mood*: The patient's general appearance, grooming, eye contact, clothing and other features can be informative. Does the patient appear his or her stated age, older, younger? A disheveled appearance is often seen in those suffering from dementia, moderate to severe depression, and schizophrenia. An unusually neat and tidy appearance may suggest obsessive-compulsive personality disorder. *Affect* is the outward emotional state of the patient observed by the clinician. Sadness, anger, happiness, and irritation are all examples of affects. Also note whether the affect is appropriate or inappropriate to the current situation and to ideation. Other parameters include the quality (flat, blunted, full, intense) and range (constricted, full, expansive). *Mood* is the sustained and reported emotion that is experienced internally by the patient. In some disorders the patient's mood is incongruent with his or her affect (i.e., a person with schizoaffective disorder who says he is extremely sad but is laughing uncontrollably). A person who is unable to identify and describe his mood state is said to have *alexythymia*.

B: *Behavior*: The patient's manner (i.e., calm, composed, agitated, or disruptive) provides added information supporting other observations regarding mood, orientation, and can yield diagnostic clues. Increased motor activity or psychomotor activation usually accompanies mania (the intensely elevated, hyperactive phase of bipolar disorder), anxiety, delirium (an acute confusional state), and/or substance intoxication (cocaine, PCP) or withdrawal (alcohol or benzodiazepines).

Decreased motor activity or psychomotor retardation occurs in depression, some types of catatonia (see Chapter 4 for the definition of catatonia), or as a side effect of medication (bradykinesia with antipsychotic usage), or substance intoxication (opioid or benzodiazepine intoxication).

S: *Speech*: Attending to the rate, volume, articulation, and fluency of the patient's speech can be a key factor in certain disorders.

T: *Thought process*: A variety of observations are made in this category. The process of the patient's thinking is important. Do his or her thoughts relate to each other logically, or do they seem random, having no bearing or relation to each other? This is called *derailment* or *loose associations*. "*The Simpsons* is my favorite TV program, I like Homer the best, the traffic lights are red and green and amber is in the middle, and Pegasus was a flying horse" is an example of loose associations from a young patient suffering from schizophrenia. To explore the process of thinking in more detail, you may ask the patient to interpret a proverb (e.g., What does it mean to say, "'Don't count your chickens before they hatch"?). If he answers concretely (e.g., "Of course, you can't count chickens until they hatch"), he may have low intelligence or dementia. If his answer is bizarre or idio-syncratic (e.g., "My chickens peek out of the egg, so you can count their beaks"), psychosis, including schizophrenia, must be considered. Other important thought process impairments to be aware of are

- *flight of ideas*: rapid and successive speech connecting unrelated ideas (often seen in mania);
- *circumstantial*: too much digression precedes communication of central idea (may be seen in schizophrenia and obsessive compulsive disorder);
- *tangential*: the speaker wanders and drifts and never returns to the original topic (may be seen in schizophrenia or very anxious patients);
- *perseveration*: an inability to move on from a particular thought or idea that is no longer appropriate to social context (may be seen in traumatic brain injury, autism, those with frontal lobe lesions);
- *thought blocking:* the inability to finish a thought, or to recall what the thought was (can be seen in schizophrenia);
- *neologisms*: new words whose meaning may be known only to the patient using it (may be seen in schizophrenia, people with brain injuries and apha-sias, and autism);
- *word salad*: incomprehensible speech consisting of words put together that have no connection (may be seen in those with dementia, schizophrenia, and occasionally in floridly manic patients);
- *clanging*: thoughts occur in sequence because of the way words sound, not because of content; they usually occur in rapid succession and may be inco-herent (may be seen in manic phase of bipolar disorder).

Another important thing to notice about a patient's thinking is thought content (see below).

R: *Reasoning and judgment*: It is important to find out whether the patient can understand acceptable patterns of behavior and consequences of his actions. This can be determined by questions like "If you found a stamped, addressed envelope in the gutter, what should you do with it?" This can help elicit whether the patient understands that such a letter should be put in a mailbox. Of course, some curious souls might pick up the letter and open it to see if there was any money in it. That's why, when you ask the question, you should say, "What should you do with it" rather than "would." In lieu of a formal question, observations about the appropriateness of the patient's behavior can be useful in evaluating judgment.

A: *Attention and memory*: This tests whether the patient can recall both distant and recent events. An example of a distant event is time and place of marriage, assuming the patient is married and not a newlywed. For short-term memory, the patient is asked to remember 3 unrelated objects and to recall them 5 minutes later. Unless the patient is very anxious, he should be able to remember 3 objects. Immediate memory is tested by asking the patient to recall digits. He should be able to repeat 6 digits forwards and 4 digits backwards. This is also a test of attention as is serial subtraction. Ask the patient to subtract 7 from 100, and to subtract 7 from that answer, etc. Trouble subtracting serial 7's occurs in delirium and dementia. With patients who have less than a high school education, try serial 3's from 50. It can also help to ask about a recent news event or to list the current and 4 previous U.S presidents. Alternatively, asking the patient to spell the word WORLD forwards, and then backwards, is an abbreviated test of concentration that is often useful.

C: *Cognition*: This includes orientation, whether the patient understands who he is, where he is, and what time it is. Patients should know the day of the week, the date, and the year. Sometimes, disorientation to time can be subtle. It may be of value to ask the patient specifically what time of the day it is or even whether he can judge when 60 seconds have elapsed. If the patient is off by more than 15 seconds, suspect disorientation. Time disorientation usually accompanies a delirium. Disorientation to place is also common in patients with a delirium. Disorientation to person is very unusual and seen only in severe central nervous system (CNS) dysfunction, amnestic states, and in some patients who are malingering. Cognition also includes intellectual functioning. This refers essentially to how well the patient can carry out calculations and other thought processes that would be commensurate with his educational level. Attention span (see above) and concentrating ability are also measured by these tasks and are diminished in delirium and dementia (often in depression, too). If his or her intellectual capabilities are diminished, this also suggests delirium, dementia, or an amnestic state. It is always important to establish the person's baseline cognitive status and compare it to the current functioning.

T: *Thought content:* What is the content of his or her thinking? Does the patient have delusions (a fixed and false belief) or paranoid ideation? Is the patient experiencing perceptual disturbances such as hallucinations (a false sensory perception not associated with real external stimuli)? If so, are they visual or auditory? Questions about suicidal and homicidal ideation should also be asked. (Please see section on suicide assessment in Chapter 3).

When presenting the findings you have gathered, it is crucial that you present the information to other health professionals in a logical, systematic, and clear way.

Assessment

A 2-sentence description of the current assessment that summarizes the patient to other health professionals is useful. The format should be:

> "This is 62 year old male with past psychiatric history of major depressive disorder and alcohol use disorder and 2 previous suicide attempts, currently being treated for increasingly depressed mood and vague suicidal ideation over the course of the last week in context of recent stressors (loss of job, argument with wife. and medication non-adherence).

In the consultation-liaison (C-L) setting, you should also include pertinent medical history in your 2-sentence summary.

Diagnosis (DSM-5)

The psychiatric diagnosis based on DSM-5 criteria.

CHAPTER 3.   THE DEPRESSED AND SUICIDAL PATIENT

Depression

Depression develops in 15-25% of the adult population at some time in life, so you can see that depression is one of the most common illnesses a physician encounters. In fact, according to the World Health Organization (WHO) global burden of disease projections, major depression and suicide will be among the 3 leading causes of morbidity and mortality worldwide by 2030.

Unfortunately, some primary-care physicians overlook this problem, allowing depression to remain untreated. The purpose of this chapter is to alert the general physician and other practitioners to the significance and clinical spectrum of depressive illness. Suicide is a frequent concomitant of depression, so we'll be discussing it too.

Theories about the etiology of depression began with the "black bile" theory of the ancient Greeks, which stated that too much bile causes changes in affect. Today's leading theories are somewhat more sophisticated versions of the ancient one. Theories that certain neurotransmitters, particularly norepinephrine and serotonin, are relatively depleted or inactivated in certain areas of the brain in patients with severe depression may seem bilious. However, they offer great promise in understanding the etiology of this illness. Depressed patients often have low levels of metabolites of serotonin and norepinephrine. Also, the fact that depressed patients occasionally have altered dexamethasone-suppressing capability (a dose of dexamethasone does not inhibit cortisol secretion the way it normally does) suggests that endocrine factors may play a role in depression. The evidence for genetic factors in the etiology of depression is strong, and the DSM-5 notes that approximately 40% of the risk may be attributed to one's genes.

Attempts at classifying the clinical syndromes or types of depression have been met with variable success. Certain dichotomies have been used to describe the ends of the depressive spectrum, but only a few are in current use. For instance, *unipolar* depression is depression alone, whereas *bipolar* depression is depression alternating with mania in bipolar I disorder, or alternating with hypomania (see Chapter 4 for descriptions) in bipolar II disorder. We think that it is most useful clinically to consider depression as occurring along a continuum of mild to severe.

Severe depression may occur anytime in the lifespan and is more common in women than in men. It is termed Major Depressive Disorder in DSM-5 if symptoms are marked and present most of the time, every day for 2 or more weeks. To meet the full criteria for this disorder the patient must have 5 of the following symptoms:

- *depressed mood or lack of interest and pleasure in life* (1 or both of these symptoms are necessary, plus at least 4 of the others below, to meet the criteria for major depression)
- *sleep disturbance* (either insomnia or excessive sleeping)
- *disturbance of appetite and/or weight* (increased or decreased)
- *marked feelings of guilt or worthlessness*
- either *persistent agitation or slowed movement*
- *poor concentration or confusion*
- *suicidal ideation or wishes to die* (or belief that life is not worth living)

Let us use our mnemonic, **ABSTRACT**, and run through a mental status examination in a severely depressed patient:

A: *Affect* is downcast, sad, and often there is a history of crying spells. Appearance is often disheveled; individuals who are usually well groomed may be surprisingly unkempt. Mood is depressed or devoid of any feeling or interest but may also be irritable.

B: *Behavior* in extremely depressed patients may show slowed movements and almost blank expressions. This is usually called *psychomotor retardation*, but if severe enough might be called *catatonia*. Highly irritable patients may appear with psychomotor agitation. Other behavioral symptoms may include a history of weight loss and decreased appetite, and disturbed sleeping (either difficulty remaining asleep or early morning awakening). Classically, the severely depressed patient awakens at 2–4 a.m. and is unable to return to sleep. Depression and anxiety are often most intense in these early morning hours. The intern gets up at 2 a.m. because her beeper goes off. She has trouble returning to sleep, because she's angry, not because she's depressed. Other behavioral symptoms include decreased sexual interest and slowed motor movements. Constipation is a classic physiological or behavioral symptom of depression.

S: *Speech* may be slow, soft, or almost monotone.

T: *Thought content* may include ideas of hopelessness or helplessness. Suicidal ideation may or may not be present. Delusional thinking, such as paranoia or believing that the patient's internal organs are rotting, may occur.

R: *Reasoning* and judgment may be impaired, particularly with respect to a patient's view that his situation is hopeless, which may lead to suicidal ideation or behavior.

A: *Attention* and memory are often impaired, especially in severe depression when patients may even appear demented. As we've noted earlier, depression must be ruled out in the evaluation of possible dementia.

C: *Cognition,* which includes orientation and intellectual functioning, may be impaired in depression.

T: *Thought process* may be coherent or disorganized.

When the diagnosis is unclear, a personal history of recurrent depression or a family history of depression or bipolar illness can help corroborate the diagnosis. Alcoholism in the patient or his or her relatives can also support the diagnosis. These are risk factors for depressive illness.

It's worth repeating that making this diagnosis is important, because depression is debilitating. Untreated depression may last 1 year or more. As many as 15% of patients with severe depression may ultimately commit suicide. Despite this, depression is an illness that responds well to appropriate treatment : 80-90% of depressed patients eventually respond to either antidepressants, cognitive behavior therapy, or electroconvulsive treatments and show a significant reduction of symptoms.

At the other end of the spectrum are the mild cases of depression. In mild depressions, judgment, orientation, intellectual functions, and memory are rarely impaired. Thought content may include ideas of self-depreciation or guilt (as in more severe depression), but extreme hopelessness or helplessness and psychotic thinking are not present. Vegetative signs also contrast with severe depression in that weight loss is unusual; weight gain is actually more common. Sleep disturbances occur at sleep onset, and psychomotor retardation is not present. Mild depression is more common in the afternoon and evening hours as opposed to the early morning hours. Constipation is unusual, but diarrhea occasionally occurs. Sexual interest is usually impaired in mild depression, too. Treatment with antidepressants is probably as effective as in severe depression, and patients more often request medications, since the newer drugs have fewer troubling side effects. Psychotherapy is often an appropriate treatment, whether the illness is mild or severe. Mild to moderate depression that does not meet the full criteria for major depressive disorder is termed *Unspecified Depressive Disorder* in DSM-5.

Chronic depression, which lasts 2 years or more, where depressed mood is present most of the day, more days than not, and includes at least 2 of the other criteria for major depressive disorder is labeled *Persistent Depressive Disorder (Dysthymia)* in DSM-5.

Substance/Medication Induced Depressive Disorder and *Depressive Disorder due to another medical condition* require criteria similar to those in the Psychoses section (Chapter 4).

To review, patients often come to psychiatrists with the simple complaint of "depression." Other frequent presenting symptoms include fatigue, crying spells, difficulty sleeping, changes in appetite or weight, and lack of interest in one's usual pursuits These are the *vegetative signs* of depression. Unfortunately, depressed patients sometimes present symptoms in confusing ways. For example, depressed children might arrive at your office with a complaint of hyperactivity or antisocial behavior. Elderly depressed patients might complain of memory impairment. Somatic complaints (lower back pain) can herald a depressive decompensation.

A number of medical illnesses figure in the differential diagnosis of depression. Among these, hypothyroidism is very common. All patients being evaluated for depression should be asked about other symptoms of hypothyroidism (cold intolerance, hair loss, weight gain). Cancer of the pancreas frequently causes depression. The reason for this is unknown. Both Addison's disease and Cushing's syndrome can cause depressive features. Certain drugs cause depression (steroids, beta blockers, interferon); even viral illness can cause patients to become depressed.

The psychiatric differential diagnosis is equally important.

1. Patients with schizophrenia feel depressed sometimes, especially several weeks to several months after their first decompensation. However, they also suffer from hallucinations, bizarre delusions, and loose associations.
2. Demented patients experience memory impairment and disorientation. Severely depressed patients can appear demented. This syndrome is called *pseudodementia*. Occasionally, dementia has to be diagnosed after a trial of antidepressant therapy has failed.
3. Bipolar patients may be floridly depressed, but also have a history of manic or hypomanic episodes.
4. Normal grief can be very difficult to distinguish from depression. Grief is such a ubiquitous and important response to loss that we will now digress and discuss it.

Grief

Grief follows the perception of a loss. Usually, the loss is a relative or close friend. People will also grieve over the loss of a limb, loss of body functioning, or loss of self-esteem (as in losing a job). Depressed people may develop their illness in the absence of an actual loss; they seem more likely to suffer vegetative signs than those who are bereaved.

There are characteristic stages in grief reactions. People who are grieving experience shock; that is, they initially feel emotionally overwhelmed by their loss. This is usually followed by anger, denial, sadness, and then some form of resolution in which the lost relative, friend, or limb is gradually given up. Grieving typically lasts for about a year.

When grief is intolerable or causes impairment it is often called complicated grief or prolonged grief. Watch out for these signs which suggest complicated grief:

1. If a surviving relative develops symptoms of the deceased relative, this is a manifestation of pathological grief. For example, a grieving widower whose wife died of colonic cancer might develop stomach aches as a sign of pathological grief.

	Depression	**Grief**
Loss	+/-	+
Thought	guilt, self-deprecation	thoughts of lost relatives/hallucinations of the deceased relative are sometimes normal. Guilt.
Timing	6-12 mos. +	1-24 mos. following a loss
Depressive Vegetative Signs	Usual	Less Common

Fig. 3-1. Depression vs grief.

2. Suicidal ideation and behavior are also on the pathological scale of grief reactions.
3. Psychosomatic reactions (ulcerative colitis, rheumatoid arthritis, etc.) and hyperactivity also are aberrant reactions of grief.
4. Grief lasting longer than 2 years is pathological.

Grieving people do feel depressed and unhappy for a period of time. In the end, the distinction between grief and depression can be difficult. In DSM-5, bereavement does not absolutely preclude the diagnosis of major depressive disorder but encourages the consideration of the entire clinical picture and cultural norms in evaluating specific clinical situations.

Suicide

The evaluation of the suicidal patient is one of the most difficult tasks faced by the psychiatrist. A patient's suicide is catastrophic for family and friends and is potentially the most devastating event that a clinician can experience. Although 15% of patients who are severely depressed may commit suicide, significant numbers of suicides occur in the absence of depression. Suicide may occur in the context of a manic episode, and bipolar patients may be as much as 15 times more likely to commit suicide in their lifetime than the general population. The setting of a suicidal act is usually one in which a person experiences intense stress. Such stress leads to affects or feelings that are completely intolerable to the patient. If the person sees no solution to the circumstances causing these intolerable affects, suicide begins to appear as "the only solution" to the situation. This is the time of *suicidal crisis* and can last a few hours to a few days. If assistance is provided, this suicidal crisis can be overcome. The patient's situation may require hospitalization or family support; the priority of this phase of the illness is to safeguard the patient.

A 3-9 month period of heightened vulnerability to suicide follows. This post-crisis phase should involve frequent monitoring of the patient. During this phase of the illness, patients' underlying problems should be treated.

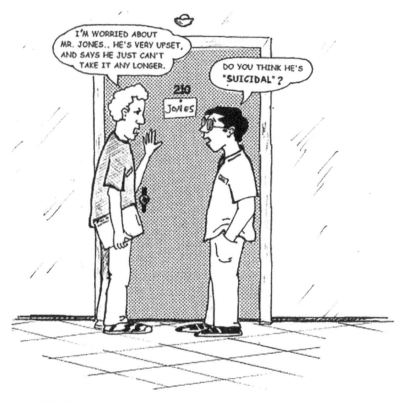

Fig. 3-2. "SUICIDAL"

For example, if they are depressed, antidepressants are usually indicated. If they have poor coping skills, efforts should be made to teach them new ways of dealing with stress.

The problem during the acute and subacute phases is how to decide the actual risk for suicide attempt. No easy answer exists, but a variety of demographic and psychological data can be elicited to help you decide. Just remember **SUICIDAL**!

S: The *Sex* of the patient is important. More men *commit* suicide; more women than men *attempt* suicide. Availability of *Significant* others is a major factor. Married patients are less likely to commit suicide than single ones, and divorced patients are at higher risk than married ones. The quality of personal relationships is also important. A patient's feelings of loneliness or isolation from important people in his or her life may lead to suicidal thinking. Part of the assessment of these relationships may include questions such as: Would you tell anyone about your plans or ideas? Would you leave a suicide note? What would it say? How do you think people would react to your death? The patient's *Spiritual*, cultural, or moral beliefs concerning death and suicide may be key factors in assessing risk.

U: *Unsuccessful* previous attempts, contrary to popular wisdom, make it more likely that an additional suicide attempt will end in death. An accurate history about previous attempts is crucial. It should include the means previously used (to assess their lethality), the presence or absence of other people at the time(s) of the attempt(s), the patient's distance from medical help at the time(s), the presence or absence of loss of consciousness, and the length of stay(s) in the hospital following the attempt(s).

I: *Identification* with family members who have committed suicide in the past may make suicide a more acceptable option to some patients. Any history of *Impulsive* behavior is important to assess.

CI: *Chronic Illness,* psychological or medical, and/or recent onset of severe illness are increased risk factors for completed suicide. Patients with depression, psychosis, chronic pain, and panic disorder are definitely at higher risk.

D: *Depression* significantly increases the risk of suicide as does *Drug* abuse.

A: The *Age* of the patient is important. A simple rule of thumb is that older men are at greater risk for suicide. Young schizophrenic males are at high risk. *Alcohol* use is also common in successful suicides. Patients acutely intoxicated with alcohol or other substance will be more impulsive and more likely to kill themselves. Chronic alcoholism is also a risk factor for suicide. It is also important to inquire about *Anniversaries* of previous traumas or the death of loved ones, since these times can lead to marked sadness and suicidal thoughts and behavior. Patients' *Alliance* or therapeutic relationship with the people who are evaluating their suicidal potential should be considered. Patients who are assessed to be most isolated and out of touch with other people are at greatest risk. Patients with suicidal ideation are very often *Ambivalent,* and this may be expressed in the interaction with the clinician whom they may see as an *Ally* if they are leaning towards living or an *Adversary* if they are truly set on dying. In these situations patients may deny any suicidal intent at all and do anything they can to avoid hospitalization or other therapeutic interventions.

L: *Lethality* of suicidal method is an important factor in the assessment. Guns, hanging, and jumping from high places are the most lethal means. Greater caution is therefore indicated with these patients. Assessing the patient's access to means they are considering is also critical, and planning means reduction (removal of guns from the home, disposing of supplies of medications, or dispensing the patient's meds by a family member for a period of time). Drug overdoses and wrist cutting are generally less lethal, but the recent increase in the availability of potent opioids has made death by drug overdose much more frequent. Recent *Losses* (death, divorce, loss of job) are also critical factors in assessing potentially suicidal patients.

Assessing suicidal potential involves the consideration of many factors. Complicating this assessment is the fact that some patients attempt suicide to manipulate "significant others." Usually, such patients are managed differently than others. It is safer, however, to assume that they are genuinely suicidal at first. If you're certain they are manipulative and don't really want to die, then hospitalization, giving in to the patients' threats, and even psychiatric treatment may not be indicated. These are tough cases, though, and consultation with a psychiatrist or psychiatric colleague is recommended before making these difficult treatment decisions.

Physicians in primary care will see the majority of depressed and suicidal patients. A significant number of patients who commit suicide have seen a doctor in the preceding several months. This suggests that they want help but can't ask for it directly. Remember **SUICIDAL** and you'll save lives!

(See Chapter 16 for treatment approaches.)

TREATMENT CONSIDERATIONS

Treatment of Depression

Medications

- Serotonin selective reuptake inhibitors (SSRIs), such as *fluoxetine* (Prozac), *paroxetine* (Paxil), *sertraline* (Zoloft), *citalopram* (Celexa), and *escitalopram* (Lexapro) are currently considered first-line treatments for major depression because of their relatively low risks of significant side effects and favorable safety profiles.
- Serotonin norepinephrine reuptake inhibitors (SNRIs), such as *venlafaxine* (Effexor); *duloxetine* (Cymbalta); and *desvenlafaxine* (Pristiq) may be considered alternative first line treatments, in certain situations, along with *bupropion* (Wellbutrin) and *mirtazapine* (Remeron). Some of these agents have a slightly greater risk of side effects such hypertension and seizures, and some experts consider them to be second-line agents in the treatment of depression.
- Tricyclic antidepressants (TCAs) and monoamine oxidase inhibitors (MAO-Is) are also very useful and important in certain clinical situations but carry a larger side effect burden, are more dangerous in overdose, and are more likely to have serious interactions with other medications and some foods.
- *Aripiprazole* (Abilify), a second-generation antipsychotic, has been approved to augment the effects of antidepressants.

(For additional specifics on medications, dosages, side effects, see Chapter 16, Treatment Modalities.)

Psychotherapy

Cognitive behavior therapy (CBT), interpersonal psychotherapy (IPT), and a number of other psychotherapy approaches including psychodynamic therapies have been shown in research studies to be significantly beneficial in major depression. Some studies have shown CBT to be comparable to medication for mild-moderate major depression. Several variations of cognitive behavior therapy, including *acceptance and commitment therapy (ACT)* and *mindfulness-based therapy* for depression, have positive research findings.

Exercise/Activity

Several research studies have suggested that a sufficient "dose" of moderate-intense exercise may have an effect comparable to antidepressants in mild-moderate major depression.

(See Chapter 16, Treatment Modalities, for definitions and discussion of various approaches to therapy and other aspects of treatment.)

ECT/TMS/DBS

Electroconvulsive therapy (ECT), in which a patient is briefly anesthetized and an electrical current is administered to the brain, inducing a seizure, is frequently effective for severe depression and may be life-saving in some cases. Often treatment is begun in an inpatient psychiatric unit, and then the patient is transitioned to outpatient ECT treatments. A typical course of ECT involves 1 treatment 3 times a week for a total of 6-10 treatments.

Transcranial magnetic stimulation (TMS) is an outpatient, noninvasive procedure, in which a magnetic field is administered to the brain. It is a newer treatment for treatment-resistant depression and may be effective in some patients. TMS is performed in a medical office setting and may consist of a 40-45 minute treatment 4-5 days a week for 4 weeks.

Deep Brain Stimulation (DBS) is actually a neurosurgical procedure in which electrodes are placed in the brain and then stimulated electrically. DBS is used most commonly in patients with Parkinson's Disease or tremors that do not respond to medication treatment, but it may be considered in patients with very severe depression who do not respond to any other form of treatment.

The above treatment types may vary depending on the following specific diagnoses:

1. *Major Depressive Disorder, mild to moderate (no psychotic symptoms and not suicidal)*

   - *Psychotherapy*: cognitive behavior therapy (CBT), interpersonal psychotherapy (IPT), other therapies, and exercise/activity; may use alone or combined with antidepressants.
   - Trial of a serotonin selective reuptake inhibitor (SSRIs — e.g., *fluoxetine, sertraline, paroxetine, citalopram, or escitalopram*) and continue therapy.
   - Titrate to usual effective dose (often 50-66% of maximum dose; e.g., 20-40mg/d of *fluoxetine* or 50-100mg/d of *sertraline*).
   - IF there is a partial response, 1st maximize dose of initial agent for 4-6 weeks, then consider different SSRI.
   - Trial of an alternative antidepressant, serotonin norepinephrine reuptake inhibitor (SNRI), e.g., *venlafaxine, duloxetine, desvenlafaxine or bupropion or mirtazapine*, IF patient has had prior unsuccessful SSRI trials.
   - An adequate medication trial is usually at least 8 weeks at effective dose of given agent.

2. *Major Depressive Disorder, moderate to severe, or partial response in patients with mild to moderate symptoms (no psychotic symptoms and not suicidal)*
   - Choices as above plus

     IF partial response, titrate to maximum dose, consider more frequent therapy.

     IF nonresponsive to initial treatment after 4-6 weeks, switch to a different antidepressant in a different class.
   - Switch with cross-taper off initial antidepressant onto 2nd drug (e.g., from *sertraline* 200mg/day to *venlafaxine XR* 225mg/day - *sertraline* 150mg/day + *venlafaxine XR* 37.5mg/day x 6 days, then *sertraline* 100mg/day + *venlafaxine XR* 75mg/day x 6 days, then *sertraline* 50mg/day + *venlafaxine XR* 150mg/day x 6 days, then discontinue *sertraline* and increase *venlafaxine XR* to 225mg/day).
   - Trial of a monoamine oxidase inhibitor (MAO-I). The patient must be off an SSRI, SNRI or TCA for at least 2 weeks before starting the MAO-I; *phenelzine* and *tranylcypromine* are most often used.
   - Consideration of a trial of repetitive Transcranial Magnetic Stimulation (rTMS).

3. *Major Depressive Disorder, moderate to severe (with psychotic symptoms or suicidal risk)*
   - Medication choices, as above.
   - Hospital admission for safety and treatment changes in protected environment.
   - Addition of an antipsychotic agent to the antidepressant; *aripiprazole* and *brexpiprazole* are FDA-approved for augmentation of antidepressants in patients with depression (with or without psychosis), but other agents may be effective as well.
   - Consideration of a trial of ECT; or, in rare cases that are refractory to multiple medications trials and ECT, DBS may be considered.

(See Chapter 16, Treatment Modalities, for further discussion of treatment options.)

CHAPTER 4. PSYCHOSES

As a busy psychiatrist, you're asked to come see a "raging, incoherent" man in the emergency room. Armed with your psychiatrist's black bag (your brain, an emergency detention form, and a pen), you're on your way to stamping out mental illness. The patient is clearly out of touch with reality, nonsensical, and loudly shouting unmentionables, and you must now figure out from what variety of psychosis he suffers.

The approach to the patient (outlined in Chapter 2) must often be modified in acute care settings. Still, it is critical that effort is made to converse with the patient, helping the patient feel that you are there and allied with him in helping him with his problems. Then you must proceed with the mental status examination (remember **ABSTRACT**).

After the mental status examination is performed, you are in a good position to categorize this patient as having a particular psychotic disorder.

Figure 4-1 is provided to help sort this out.

Although the mental status examination is most helpful in diagnosing these various conditions, other information is also of value.

While psychotic symptoms may briefly occur in patients with many psychiatric disorders, florid and persistent psychosis occurs most commonly in the conditions we will consider now.

Schizophrenia

No psychiatric disorder is more disabling than schizophrenia. The term schizophrenia has been misused to describe patients with "split personalities." Schizophrenia actually refers to a very specific psychotic illness. In DSM-5, schizophrenia is now in the section entitled "Schizophrenia Spectrum and Other Psychotic Disorders." These disorders are characterized by symptoms in related categories: delusions, hallucinations, disorganized thinking, disorganized or catatonic behavior, or negative symptoms. The diagnosis of schizophrenia is made if the patient has 2 or more of the above symptoms for much of the time over a 1-month period, major areas of functioning in life are affected, and the illness persists with some significant symptoms for over 6 months. To fulfill criteria for schizophrenia, the

	A appearance, affect/mood	B behavior	S speech	T thought process	R reason/ judgment	A attention/ memory	C cognition	T thought content
Schizophrenia	disheveled appearance, flat affect, inappropriate to content of speech	variable	normal to disorganized	normal to very disorganized, loose associations	poor	usually normal	usually normal	delusions, auditory hallucinations
Mania	mood euphoric, irritable, or expansive; affect intense	flamboyant dress, motor activity	speech pressured	racing thoughts, flight of ideas	poor	may be normal, or impaired due to flight of ideas	may be normal, or impaired due to flight of ideas	grandiosity, delusional
Dementia	affect may be depressed, labile, or inappropriate	may be unkempt and unaware	normal, or poverty of speech	perseveration, loose associations	poor	poor memory & attention	disoriented to time and place, rarely to person	+/- paranoia, delusions hallucinations
Delusional Disorder	appearance OK, affect may be normal or suspicious	may be normal or suspicious	normal	normal, except regarding delusion	normal, except regarding delusion	normal	normal	delusional, may try to conceal
Delirium	affect and mood variable	variable, may be agitated	variable	may be disorganized may be quiet, cautious	poor	memory impaired attention very poor	disoriented to time & place, rarely to person	may have hallucinations usually visual

Fig. 4-1.   ABSTRACT comparison of psychiatric disorders.

	Age of onset	Type Hallucination	Family History
Bipolar Disorder	20-40	Usually Auditory	Usually +
Schizophrenia	15-30	Usually Auditory	Sometimes +
Delirium/Dementia	Any age	Usually Visual	Rarely +

Fig. 4-2.   Additional data to help corroborate the above psychiatric diagnoses.

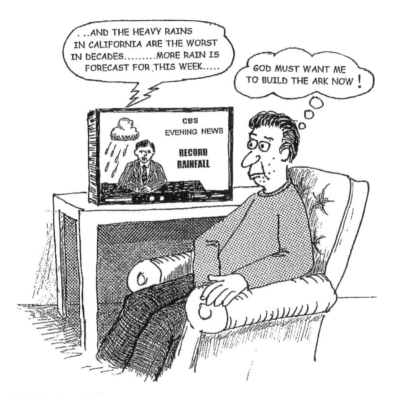

Fig. 4-3.   Ideas of reference.

individual must have at least 1 of the following 3 "positive" symptoms: delusions, hallucinations, or disorganized speech. *Negative symptoms* may be thought of as a loss of normal functioning, including a loss of motivation (*avolition*), a loss of the ability to express emotion (*affective flattening*), a loss of the ability to generate speech (*alogia*), or a loss of the ability to experience joy or pleasure (*anhedonia*).

A feeling that the television is personally communicating with the patient, and the feeling that the patient's thoughts are being controlled by someone else are examples of schizophrenic delusions.

The age of onset of schizophrenia is usually late adolescence to early adulthood. The patient's age can be useful diagnostically when the mental status examination is ambiguous. Although the diagnostic findings above are most valid in distinguishing schizophrenia from other psychoses, there are additional diagnostic criteria. Eugen Bleuler, a Swiss psychiatrist, coined the term *schizophrenia* and described some of the key phenomenology, the 4-A's, at the turn of the 20th century. The 4-A's stand for:

- *Autism*: Idiosyncratic ideas and attitudes.
- *Associations*: The schizophrenic patient has loose associations (remember Pegasus in the example of loose associations in Chapter 2?).
- *Ambivalence*: *Ambivalence* refers to an inability on the patient's part to make up his or her mind. In the extreme, ambivalence may cause paralysis of action, i.e., catatonia. For example, the patient stands in a doorway for hours, unable to decide whether to enter or leave.
- *Affect*: The affect in schizophrenic patients is typically "flat" (diminished intensity) or inappropriate to the content of their speech.

Except for the loose associations, these 4-As comprise most of the symptoms currently described as "negative symptoms" of schizophrenia.

It's not uncommon for patients suffering from schizophrenia to have co-occurring substance use disorders (nicotine, alcohol, sedatives, marijuana, etc.). Needless to say, this can cloud the diagnostic picture. Individuals with chronic schizophrenia often have fixed delusional symptoms that serve as their basic orientation to the world. They may have little apparent anxiety and maintain that they have no problems at all; it's just that the FBI has some special mission for them—that's the problem.

One other aspect of schizophrenia bears mentioning. *Catatonia* is an accompanying feature in some schizophrenic patients. Catatonia refers to a disorder both of motor control and speech that develops in several conditions. In schizophrenia, *waxy flexibility* (patient maintains an enforced posture) and mutism are features of catatonia. Occasionally, agitated catatonia can develop. This type of catatonia is characterized by extreme psychomotor agitation and requires emergency psychiatric intervention, either in the form of rapid tranquilization or electroconvulsive therapy (ECT). We'll have more to say about these forms of treatment later.

The risk of suicide is high in schizophrenia, especially in male patients under 30. Depression and suicidal ideation should be evaluated and often require hospitalization.

In DSM-5, schizophrenia is no longer classified according to the predominant symptomatology (disorganized, paranoid, catatonic, and undifferentiated in DSM-IV). The only additional specifiers that may be used are: number of episodes, first episode, multiple episodes or continuous; level of remission (if applicable), acute episode, in partial remission, in full remission; or, with catatonia (if present).

A diagnosis of *Brief Psychotic Disorder* is made in a person with symptoms of schizophrenia but requires that the symptoms last at least 1 day and less than 1 month with eventual return to full pre-morbid functioning. The symptom profile of *Schizophreniform Disorder* is identical to that of schizophrenia; however, the total duration of illness must be less than 6 months. Also, a deterioration in social or occupational functioning, which is required to make the diagnosis, is not required for schizophreniform disorder. About 70% of those diagnosed with schizophreniform disorder are later diagnosed with schizophrenia.

Schizoaffective Disorder

Patients with this disorder meet the criteria for a major mood disorder (depression or mania) while at the same time meeting criteria for schizophrenia during a period of at least 2 weeks during the illness. At other times during the illness they must have delusions or hallucinations for at least 2 weeks without major mood symptoms; however, over time, symptoms of a major mood episode must be present the majority of time over the course of the illness.

Delusional (Paranoid) Disorder

A circumscribed delusion or delusional system lasting 1 month or longer, with other mental functioning spared (i.e., criteria for schizophrenia are not met), characterizes *Delusional Disorder*. This disorder presents in adulthood and may not come to the psychiatrist's attention. Such patients are often adept at keeping their delusions secret. A key change in DSM-5 (from DSM - IV - TR) is that delusions are no longer required to be "non – bizarre". The DSM - 5 retains the types of delusional disorder: *erotomanic*, *grandiose*, *jealous*, *persecutory*, *somatic*, and *unspecified*. Acute and chronic forms exist, the latter being more difficult to treat. Persecutory beliefs (*paranoia*) can be a symptom of other illnesses, including schizophrenia, severe depression, and drug ingestion.

People with *paranoid personality disorders* are extremely suspicious or jealous but do not have delusions.

Substance-Induced Psychotic Disorder and Psychotic Disorder Due to Another Medical Condition

These disorders (as defined in DSM-5) are diagnosed in patients with delusions and/or hallucinations and in whom there is evidence the onset of symptoms is related to a substance/medication or a general medical condition. While these conditions are related to patients with a delirium (see below), they are defined by symptoms that do not occur exclusively in the course of a delirium.

TREATMENT CONSIDERATIONS

Medications

Second-Generation Antipsychotics

These agents are now used first-line by most practitioners for treatment of psychotic disorders: *olanzapine, quetiapine, risperidone, aripiprazole, ziprazidone, lurasidone, iloperidone, brexpiprazole* and *asenapine*. *Clozapine* is used primarily for illness refractory to usual treatment due to the risk of agranulocytosis.

First-Generation Antipsychotics

These agents are considered second-line treatment by most clinicians, with noted exceptions: *haloperidol* (often used IM for acute agitation in inpatient settings), *perphenazine, fluphenazine, chlorpromazine, trifluoperazine, loxapine,* and others.

Psychosocial Treatments

- Intensive case management
- Supported housing, individual apartments or group homes
- Sheltered work programs
- Cognitive behavior therapy

The above treatment considerations may vary, depending on the following specific diagnoses:

Treatment of Schizophrenia, first episode or relapse (not suicidal, not agitated or in urgent need of hospital admission):

- Second-generation antipsychotic (SGA), oral preparation.
- Choose an agent that targets the patient's most troubling symptoms (e.g., *olanzapine* and *quetiapine* are more sedating and may help patients with marked insomnia, whereas *aripiprazole, ziprasidone* and *lurasidone* may be more effective in patients with marked apathy and withdrawal).
- Typical starting dosages:
  olanzapine 2.5-5mg daily titrating to 10mg daily over about 2 weeks, maximum 20mg daily
  quetiapine 25-50mg daily titrating to 300-500mg daily over about 2 weeks, maximum 750mg daily.
- First-generation antipsychotics (FGAs) are used less frequently today; however, one major recent research study suggested *perphenazine* may have similar efficacy and safety to newer agents.
- Typical starting dosage:
  perphenazine 2-4mg tid, titrating to 24-32mg daily over about 2 weeks, maximum 64mg daily
- The medical adage "start low and go slow" is especially important in these patients as treatment adherence is correlated with experience of adverse effects, which is often related to dose escalation; therefore, treatment and dose titration must be individualized.

Treatment of Schizophrenia, first episode or relapse (agitated, suicidal or otherwise dangerous, in hospital or in need of same):

- SGA, in orally disintegrating tablet or liquid form (e.g., *olanzapine, risperidone,* or *aripiprazole*) if patient accepts oral medications.

- Or, short-acting IM (e.g., *olanzapine, aripiprazole* or *ziprasidone*); starting dosages are roughly equivalent to oral formulation, but titration is more rapid, usually achieving target dose within 2-3 days.
- First-generation antipsychotic (FGA), short-acting IM *haloperidol* (often combined with IM *lorazepam*) has been used as the mainstay of acute treatment in agitated psychotic patients.
- Goal is to stabilize patients with minimal psychotic symptoms and maximum functionality to facilitate opportunity for recovery.

Treatment of Schizophrenia, maintenance treatment:
- Oral SGAs, whichever agent is most tolerable to the patient, are most commonly prescribed for maintenance; however, long-acting injectable SGAs *(risperidone, aripiprazole, olanzapine* or *paliperidone)* or FGAs *(haloperidol* or *fluphenazine)* have been shown to reduce relapse and hospital admission rates in patients with chronic schizophrenia.

Treatment of Schizophrenia, refractory:
- *Clozapine* has been shown to produce significant reductions in psychotic symptoms and similar improvements in function, leading toward recovery in many patients with minimal response to other medications.
- Electroconvulsive therapy (ECT) is often very effective in patients with schizophrenia who are catatonic or markedly agitated and unresponsive to other treatments.
- Psychosocial treatments, including intensive case management, supported housing, sheltered work programs, and cognitive behavior therapy, are helpful for many patients with schizophrenia.

(See Chapter 16, Treatment Modalities, for further discussion of treatment options.)

CHAPTER 5.   BIPOLAR DISORDER

Bipolar Disorder is a curious yet common disorder (the lifetime prevalence of Bipolar I is 1%) of mood and affect regulation, which usually begins in the patient's late teens to early 20's, but occasionally patients are seen with later onset. The illness involves periodic episodes of either severe mania or severe depression, although the basic requirement to meet criteria for Bipolar I is at least 1 manic episode (depressive episodes are not required for the diagnosis of Bipolar I).

Manic episodes develop rapidly over the course of a few hours to a few days and can last 3-4 months without treatment. A manic episode is defined as a discrete period of elevated, expansive, or irritable mood accompanied by a high level of energy or activity lasting a minimum of 1 week and including at least 3 (or 4 if the mood is only irritable) other symptoms:

- decreased need for sleep (feels rested after 3 hours sleep, or less)
- increased goal-directed activity or psychomotor activity
- distractibility
- grandiosity (which may be delusional), euphoria, or markedly elevated self esteem
- extreme talkativeness or pressure of speech
- racing thoughts (subjective experience) or flight of ideas (including frank psychosis)
- preoccupation with activities that are high risk and uncharacteristic of the person when mood is normal, e.g., sexual indiscretions, financial schemes

The disruption in a manic episode is so severe that the person is markedly impaired and may be psychotic and may require psychiatric hospitalization.

The criteria for a hypomanic episode is that it must last at least 4 days and have at least 3 of the symptoms of a manic episode (4 if the mood is irritable). Basically a hypomanic episode is less intense than a manic episode, does not cause marked impairment or psychosis and the patient does not require hospital admission.

Generally, depressive episodes last from 3–8 months (provided no treatment is implemented) and may be interspersed with periods of relatively healthy adult functioning.

Depressive episodes are characterized by symptoms over a minimum of 2 weeks, including markedly depressed mood OR anhedonia (lack of interest and pleasure) and at least 4 of the following:

- appetite or weight changes (increased or decreased)
- disturbed sleep (insomnia or hypersomnia)
- psychomotor retardation or agitation
- decreased energy
- decreased concentration
- feelings of guilt or worthlessness
- suicidal thinking or wishes to die

Bipolar II disorder is characterized by a history of at least 1 hypomanic episode and 1 major depressive episode but no history of a manic episode.

In fact, many people with Bipolar disorder actually function at a hypomanic level (very energetic but not fully in a manic phase) and can get extraordinary amounts of work and chores done. Eventually, though, many patients will enter a manic phase, which is characterized by the euphoria, pressured speech, extreme motor hyperactivity, sleeplessness, social intrusiveness, and other symptoms enumerated above. When such patients enter a depressive phase, which actually occurs much more commonly than the manic phase, the reverse is true. A depressed mood, decreased motor activity, retarded speech, hyposexuality, and sleep disturbance may be the cardinal symptoms of a depressive phase.

The *elevated mood* seen in mania can be quite difficult to recognize. Most often, these patients are also irritable. When prevented from doing something that they have their mind set on, they can react with both irritation and angry outbursts. Sometimes lacunae of depressive mood accompany the elevated mood.

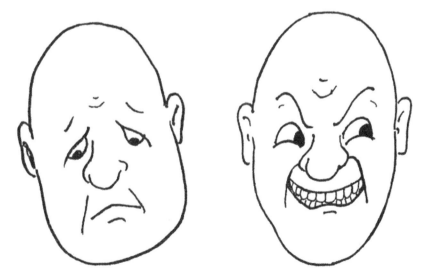

Fig. 5-1.   Bipolar disorder. Same person, different weeks (or months).

	Olfactory	Auditory	Visual	Tactile
Illness	Temporal lobe seizures Tumor, stroke, trauma	Usually Schizophrenia or Bipolar	Delirium Hallucinogens Brain tumor Migraine Dementia with Lewy Bodies	Cocaine abuse (formication) Delirium tremens

Fig. 5-2.   The differential diagnosis of hallucinations.

Pressured speech, not dissimilar from the speech of someone who has abused amphetamines or recently drunk ten cups of coffee, is characterized by sensical but fast and loud locution. In its extreme form, pressured speech is sometimes termed *flight of ideas.* Generally, a bipolar patient will make sense to an interviewer, whereas a schizophrenic often seems nonsensical (although sometimes the distinction is difficult).

Hyperactivity is a relatively nonspecific psychiatric symptom. Motor outlets for feelings are commonly employed by children, but are also seen in anxious and bipolar adults. An inability to sit still, constant crossing and recrossing of the legs, and fidgeting with arms and hands may be the outward manifestation of this aspect of the illness. Sleeplessness is almost always present in mania.

In addition to these cardinal symptoms, a variety of other problems can accompany bipolar illness. Typically, the history of these patients reveals that they have been spending money wildly. Although this behavior is characteristic of the housestaff who have recently graduated and entered private practice, it is abnormal when the patient reports having no money or is delusional about how much money he or she has. A loss of touch with reality is almost always present to some degree and can be accompanied by frank delusions, usually of a grandiose nature, and hallucinations. Hallucinations are interesting phenomena and can be very useful when trying to distinguish various kinds of disorders.

Here are some other important facts about Bipolar Disorder: males and females are equally affected, as are people of all socioeconomic and racial/ethnic backgrounds; suicide risk is high, almost 20%; 50% of Bipolar I patients have psychotic symptoms at some point; up to 80% of patients had substance use problems; and episodes may recur indefinitely.

In DSM-5, Bipolar Spectrum Disorders include Bipolar I, Bipolar II, Cyclothymia, Substance/Medication-Induced Bipolar Disorder, Bipolar Disorder Due to Another Medical Condition, Other Specified Bipolar Disorder, and Unspecified Bipolar Disorder.

TREATMENT CONSIDERATIONS

Medications

Lithium was the first effective medication for bipolar disorder and officially approved for this use by the FDA in 1970. It is still considered by many experienced clinicians as the first-line bipolar medication. It is possibly most effective in patients with euphoric mania. Recent research may lead to specific genes that indicate lithium responsiveness.

Anticonvulsants (*divalproex*, *carbamazepine*, and *lamotrigine*) have also been approved for bipolar disorder. These agents may be most effective in patients with comorbid drug abuse, mania where irritable mood is predominant, or mixed manic states.

Most *second-generation antipsychotics* have also been approved for use in bipolar disorder, and may be particularly helpful in acute mania. In addition, 3 of these agents, *quetiapine*, *lurasidone* (in combination with lithium or valproate), or *olanzapine* (combined with the antidepressant *fluoxetine*) have been approved for the treatment of bipolar depression. *Clozapine* may be effective in refractory cases.

Psychosocial Treatments

Psychoeducation of patients and families concerning the illness and course of treatment has compared favorably with cognitive behavior therapy in some studies. Cognitive Behavior Therapy (CBT) has been shown, in some studies, to be effective in reducing relapse risk in bipolar disorder, possibly by improving medication adherence and alleviating depressive symptoms.

Electro-Convulsive Therapy (ECT) may be life-saving in certain cases.

The above treatment considerations may vary depending on the following specific diagnoses:

Treatment of Bipolar I Disorder, Manic Phase:

- Acute mania often requires inpatient psychiatric admission to stop or prevent the continuation or recurrence of dangerous and/or costly impulsive behaviors.
- A mood stabilizer is essential in practically all cases. *Lithium* has the most evidence for efficacy, and is particularly useful in patients with euphoric mania (more recent research points to specific genetic markers in bipolar patients most likely to respond to lithium).
- Typical starting dose of *lithium* is 300mg tid or 450mg bid, then titrating to a target blood level of 0.8-1.2 mEq/L within 1 week.
- *Valproate* (including *divalproex* and *valproic acid*) is another mood stabilizer that may be most useful in bipolar I patients with mixed mania and depression and/or drug and alcohol abuse.
- Typical starting dose of *valproate* is 500mg bid titrating to a valproic acid blood level of 80-100 mcg/mL.
- *Carbamazepine* is the 3rd mood stabilizer that is often considered a foundation for maintenance treatment of bipolar disorder. This agent is not often useful in acute mania as it must be titrated slowly to effective maintenance dose due to the risk of rare but serious side effects, including severe skin rash or aplastic anemia.
- Second-generation antipsychotics (SGAs) are considered "mood stabilizers" because they have FDA indications for bipolar disorder as well as for

schizophrenia. In most cases they should be considered secondary agents, useful for acute agitation and psychotic symptoms.

- The first-generation antipsychotic (FGA) *haloperidol* (used IM, and often along with *lorazepam*) is frequently used in inpatient settings for acute agitation.
- Electroconvulsive therapy (ECT) is at times necessary to stabilize a patient with severe mania.
- Several weeks are often required to completely stabilize a patient who has had an acute manic episode.

Treatment of Bipolar I Disorder, Depressed Phase:

- Inpatient hospital admission is required in some cases.
- A mood stabilizer is recommended in all patients with bipolar I disorder, including those with recurrent depressive episodes, although some patients feel the drug may contribute to the depressed mood. *Lamotrigine* should be added to the treatments for this phase of the illness as it has been shown to delay the recurrence of depressive episodes. It is less effective in manic or mixed episodes.
- Second-generation antipsychotics (*quetiapine*, *lurasidone* and *olanzapine* [in combination with *fluoxetine*]) have FDA indications for bipolar depression and are widely used today.
- Antidepressant use in the depressed phase of this disorder is controversial. Some evidence supports the view that patients' mood cycles are more frequent when an antidepressant is added. This is especially true with tricyclic antidepressants but may be less so with newer agents.

Treatment of Bipolar II Disorder:

- As most of these patients present in the depressed phase, the treatment is similar to that of patients with bipolar I, depressed; that is, use a mood stabilizer such as *lamotrigine* or one of the SGAs noted above.
- Maintenance treatment in all phases of these disorders is most effective with continuation of the medication that facilitated resolution of the mood episode.

(See Chapter 16, Treatment Modalities, for further discussion of treatment options.)

CHAPTER 6. DELIRIUM/DEMENTIA

The patient with *delirium* or *dementia* (now termed *Major Neurocognitive Disorder* in DSM-5) may present as clinically psychotic. The principal manifestations of dementia are memory impairment with no disturbance in the level of consciousness (unless delirium is also present) plus other cognitive difficulties (specifically apraxia [inability to carry out movements despite an intact motor system], agnosia [inability to recognize or identify objects], or aphasia [language disturbance]). *Perseveration,* repeating of the same words or phrases, also can develop.

Disorientation to time and other changes in the level of consciousness occurring acutely are the hallmarks of a delirium; disorientation to place and, rarely, person may occur in later stages. Delirium goes by many other names, including *altered mental status, encephalopathy,* and *acute brain syndrome.* Dementia develops gradually, and patients often have time to attempt to compensate for their impaired cognitive functioning. When acute confusion (delirium) occurs in a patient with dementia, anxiety and even depression can accompany the disorder.

A delirium is usually reversible, but dementia is usually not reversible. Delirium may be worse at night. This is termed *sundowning.*

Delirium and dementia are symptoms secondary to underlying medical conditions. There are multiple causes for these syndromes; therefore, a systematic approach to the patient is necessary to ensure the discovery of the disorder's cause, as both are treatable, and certain types of dementia are actually reversible.

Can a person with an isolated small stroke develop a dementia? Do patients with brain tumors develop the manifestations of delirium? The answer to these questions is usually "no." To develop delirium or dementia, the patient must be suffering from CNS (central nervous system) disease that affects both cerebral hemispheres. Usually, a stroke affects one area of the brain. If the stroke causes extensive edema, then both hemispheres could be affected. Likewise, a brain tumor won't result in dementia or delirium unless it's very diffuse or very large (large enough to impinge on both cerebral hemispheres). Of course, specific neurologic deficits will accompany punctate lesions in the central nervous system, but memory impairment and disorientation usually occur in the company of diffuse CNS disease. Knowing that, let's explore the types of disorders that can cause these problems.

The most common types of dementia are *Alzheimers Dementia* (60+%), *Vascular Dementia* (~15%), and *Dementia with Lewy Bodies* (~15%). Other categories of dysfunction include:

- *Endocrine disorders*: In the more severe stages of these diseases, endocrine dysfunction affects the entire body, as well as the entire brain. Disorders such as hypothyroidism, Addison's disease, ketoacidosis, and hypoglycemia can cause a delirium or in some cases a reversible dementia.
- *Drug ingestions*: Since drugs are systemically distributed, many drugs can cause a delirium (e.g., ethanol, barbiturates, hallucinogens, anticholinergics, steroids), but chronic use, especially of ethanol, may lead to a dementia that is at times reversible. Drug withdrawal, especially of ethanol or benzodiazepines, but occasionally other drugs, may precipitate a delirium, including the potentially fatal *delirium tremens*.
- *Metabolic conditions*: Liver failure, renal failure, heart failure, respiratory failure, and significant serum and electrolyte abnormalities would be expected to affect the entire brain and, therefore, are occasionally responsible for the development of delirium.
- *Infections*: Any infection that involves the entire brain would be expected to cause a delirium. Meningitis and encephalitis occasionally present in this fashion. HIV is another potentially reversible cause of the syndrome of dementia. How about a brain abscess? Actually a brain abscess would cause focal neurologic findings; it would cause these disorders only if it were huge, causing swelling or compression of most of the brain.
- *Intrinsic CNS disease*: Large brain tumors, massive strokes, and head trauma do occasionally present as a dementia. More typically, these disorders present in other ways. *Arteriosclerotic brain disease* is frequently cited as a cause for dementia (vascular dementia). However, *only* patients with multiple, small infarcts affecting large areas of the brain are prone to develop a dementia.

When does a delirium become a dementia and vice versa? There is no easy answer to this question. Some forms of brain insult are irreversible, while others are quite readily reversed. In general, the quicker the diagnosis is made and the faster the underlying medical condition is reversed, the better the prognosis. These syndromes can present at all ages. By the way, a 65-year-old man presenting with acute onset of bizarre delusions and hallucinations would not have schizophrenia, because that illness is never seen developing at this age. As you have noted from the hallucination chart, visual hallucinations are most commonly seen in delirium or other specific brain disorder such as Lewy Body Dementia. This is frequently a helpful distinguishing factor.

For teaching purposes, we have simplified the nomenclature for delirium and dementia. The above schema should serve you well in diagnosing most of these conditions, but please remember that exceptions exist:

1. If your patient has had a personality change, but still has intact memory and orientation, suspect a brain disorder. An example of this would be a conservative businessman who begins acting radically because he has a frontal lobe tumor.

2. Delusional patients may be suffering from an ingestion, especially of co-caine, amphetamines, caffeine, hallucinogens, or steroids. Memory and orientation could be spared in this case, although the cause is substance induced.
3. Selected stroke syndromes and drugs (e.g., amphetamines, steroids, reser-pine) can cause mood disorders.
4. Hallucinations can be caused by organic conditions. Sometimes memory and orientation are not affected.

Now we return to that wild and agitated patient whom you were called to see at the beginning of this chapter. With your mental status exam and knowledge of the major forms of psychosis, you are able to pin down the diagnosis. Unfortunately, with these kinds of patients, your life is usually not so simple as walking into the examining room and taking a careful history. Some of these patients are agitated and combative and would most likely take a swing at you, if you were not careful. Therefore, in conducting your interview and evaluation, it's important to make sure that you, yourself, are safe and that your patient is protected from himself. So, if you have to go see a patient like this, be sure to have a hospital security guard or 2 accompany you, and be sure not to let the patient head for the hills. We'll have more on the treatment of these disorders later.

TREATMENT CONSIDERATIONS

The treatment of delirium or dementia follows the diagnosis of the cause of the condition of course. In the case of a general medical condition such as a systemic infection or hypothyroidism, the treatment is focused on the precipitating disorder. Judicious use of benzodiazepines or antipsychotics may be beneficial.

(See Chapter 16, Treatment Modalities, for further discussion of treatment options.)

CHAPTER 7.   THE ANXIOUS PATIENT

Most physicians don't respond to a request for an antianxiety medication by reaching for their prescription pads, but a systematic approach to the problem of anxiety is a difficult task. Anxiety is a prominent symptom in many psychiatric and medical disorders. Anxiety can also be a perfectly normal response that accompanies frightening or distressing situations. For example, examinations arouse anxiety! We would like to provide you with a method to systematically approach the problem of anxiety, so you won't be nervous the next time an anxious patient enters your office.

Anxiety cannot be quantified. It's a subjective symptom comprised of the moods of apprehension and worry. It also has physiological components of motor tension and autonomic hyperactivity. Anxiety occurs either "spontaneously" (primary), secondary to other psychiatric conditions; or secondary to medical disease. For the sake of this discussion, we'll consider anxiety about the National Boards (or other strong stimuli) to be normal (whew!), unless the anxiety results in avoidance behavior or a panic attack that does not allow a person to complete the exam. If you skip the test, or if your hand is shaking so hard that you can't write answers to the questions, that's a problem.

Deciding what constitutes normal versus pathological anxiety can be difficult. Let patients tell you how distressed they feel. Understanding the individual's subjective experience of anxiety is important. Look for behavioral changes designed to avoid anxiety, such as staying at home all day instead of going to work. Your subjective impression of normal and abnormal behavior is also important. Try to judge whether the anxiety is appropriate to the situation.

Be aware, too, that patients may not complain of anxiety per se. Complaints of lightheadedness, tingling in extremities, hyperventilation, and a sense of "unreality" are often expressions of anxiety.

Primary Anxiety Disorders

Primary Anxiety conditions include panic disorder, agoraphobia, specific phobia, social anxiety disorder (social phobia), and generalized anxiety disorder. Nearly 30% percent of the population will develop an anxiety disorder in their lifetime, and 75% of individuals diagnosed with an anxiety disorder will have their first episode in their early 20s.

Phobias are persistent, intense, and disabling fears that are out of proportion to actual danger.

Examples of specific phobias include animals, environments, blood, places, and situations.

Agoraphobia is the fear or avoidance of certain situations, like riding a bus, being in crowded areas (or open areas), or being outside of the home alone because of thoughts that say, "I won't be able to escape this situation if I suffer a panic attack or some other embarrassing or incapacitating symptoms."

Social Anxiety Disorder (Social Phobia) is the fear of embarrassment or humiliation in a public setting.

Panic Disorder refers to panic attacks that usually occur out of the clear blue and result in transient, acute, and severe anxiety. Patients with this condition eventually get anxious about becoming anxious and begin doing things in order to avoid panic attacks (e.g., staying in the house all the time). The panic attacks can't be due to another medical condition or substance use. The specifier *with panic attacks* is added to any DSM-5 diagnosis and can arise from a calm or an anxious state. This specifier is crucial to note in a patient's chart because it can be used as a marker for prognosis or severity of a particular diagnosis.

Some people are anxious all the time. They manifest a sort of hyper-vigilance and autonomic hyper-arousal. This is known as *Generalized Anxiety Disorder*

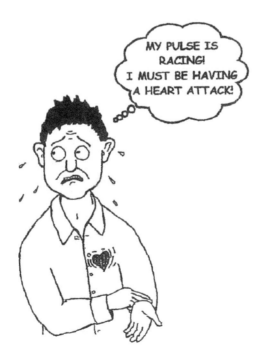

Fig. 7-1. Generalized anxiety; panic attack.

(GAD), which is likely accompanied by increased sweating, palpitations, apprehension, the feeling that "something" bad might happen, or anxiety. GAD patients often have co-occurring psychiatric conditions, especially mood disorders. The cause of GAD is unknown, but psychotherapy (CBT, psychodynamic or supportive psychotherapy) with or without antianxiety medication is the treatment of choice.

Anxiety Secondary to Psychiatric Disease

Certain psychiatric conditions are notorious for generating intense amounts of anxiety. First, and foremost, is schizophrenia. The feeling of losing one's mind, hearing voices, or having delusions is extremely frightening. Antipsychotic medications are not specifically antianxiety, but they do help dampen the distress.

When people suffering from dementia realize that their memory is failing, they may suffer what is called a *catastrophic reaction*. Enormous amounts of anxiety and panic accompany the utter incomprehension associated with this illness. Anxiety can accompany delirium, too. About 30-40% percent of people with depression suffer from anxiety.

Anxiety Secondary to Another Medical Condition

Some medical conditions cause anxiety and should figure into the differential diagnosis. Consequently, anyone reporting significant anxiety should receive a thorough history and physical exam. Appropriate labs and testing should be obtained, such as routine vitals, comprehensive metabolic panel, complete blood count, urinalysis, glucose levels, thyroid panel, troponin levels, urinary drug screen, and ECG. As a general rule, anxiety due to another medical condition can present like any of the psychiatric manifestations of anxiety (e.g., dissociative episodes, generalized anxiety, panic attacks, etc.).

First, consider the possibility that drugs may be causing the problem (either intoxication or withdrawal). Anticholinergics can cause anxiety (antipsychotics, tricyclics, etc.). as can nicotine, amphetamines, cocaine, and coffee. Sedative-hypnotics occasionally induce paradoxical arousal and anxiety. Alcohol and sedative-hypnotic withdrawals typically cause restlessness, anxiety, and elevated vital signs. Hallucinogens can also cause anxiety, because the perceptual changes that they induce may be frightening.

If drugs are not involved, then move on to common medical problems. Hyperthyroidism can cause agitation and anxiety. Hypoglycemia can induce anxiety symptoms, since it causes secretion of epinephrine. Cardiac arrhythmias occasionally cause nervousness. Hypoxia also makes people nervous and agitated.

Still no luck? Then it's time to consider the rare birds (**Fig. 7-2**). *Pheochromocytomas* secrete catecholamines, which cause intermittent symptoms of anxiety. *Acute intermittent porphyria, insulinomas* (by causing hypoglycemia), *carcinoid tumors*, and even *temporal lobe epilepsy* have been implicated in anxiety symptoms.

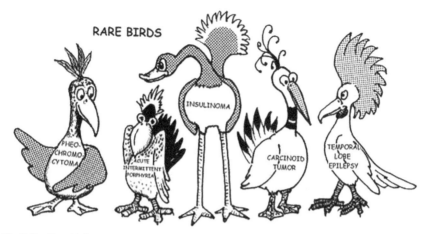

RARE BIRDS

PHEO-CHROMO-CYTOMA

ACUTE INTERMITTENT PORPHYRIA

INSULINOMA

CARCINOID TUMOR

TEMPORAL LOBE EPILEPSY

Fig. 7-2. Rare birds.

Finally, don't forget that anyone who is ill may feel nervous about the illness. Although this should be considered normal situational anxiety, it may be an indication for treatment. For example, patients immediately after myocardial infarction may need antianxiety treatment to help prevent the development of arrhythmias. Agitated, anxious patients may also need medication if they are in traction, need to be still, or are suffering significant psychological distress.

Obsessive-Compulsive and Related Disorders

Obsessive-compulsive traits are seen in anxious people who try to squelch their anxiety by thinking or performing rituals. Obsessive-compulsive traits are common in many people, especially physicians. Such traits are normal, unless physicians feel they must check their doctor's orders form a hundred times before leaving the hospital. In that case they have *obsessive-compulsive disorder*. Do not confuse *obsessive-compulsive personality disorder (OCPD)*, which is ego-syntonic (thoughts, feelings and beliefs that are in keeping with the individual's internal image of herself), with obsessive-compulsive disorder, which is ego-dystonic (the opposite of ego-syntonic, i.e., thoughts, feelings or beliefs an individual has which feel alien or incompatible with his or her internal self-image). OCPD is characterized by a perfectionistic lifestyle and the need for control over all aspects of one's lifestyle. To diagnose OCD, there must be obsessions followed by compulsions, and the symptoms must cause significant distress and total 1 hour or more per day.

- *Obsessions* are recurrent and intrusive thoughts, feelings, ideas, or sensations that increase anxiety.
- *Compulsions* are conscious, standardized, recurring patterns of behavior to relieve the anxiety of the obsession.

There are several related disorders:

- *Body dysmorphic disorder:* Individuals are preoccupied with an imagined deficit in appearance. The preoccupation may involve staring at their reflection incessantly, trying to seek continual reassurance from others, or excessive grooming. Patients imagine that they are ugly, and the preoccupation typically centers around 1 aspect of the body but can also involve several areas over time. These patients may repeatedly go to the dermatologist or seek out repeated cosmetic surgery.
- *Hoarding disorder:* These individuals acquire too many possessions and have great difficulty discarding or getting rid of them when they are no longer useful or needed. This behavior becomes a disorder when the clutter and disorganization interfere with their health or safety (exits in the home are blocked) or lead to significant distress. Simply collecting or owning lots of things does not qualify as hoarding.
- *Trichotillomania (Hair-Pulling Disorder)* results in a noticeable area of hair loss; the individual has attempted to stop or decrease the behavior in the past but is unable to do so.
- *Excoriation (Skin-Picking) Disorder* results in skin lesions; the individual has attempted to stop or decrease the behavior in the past but can't.

Post-traumatic Stress and Related Disorders

When individuals have been exposed to a severely stressful event that involves actual or threatened death, serious injury, or sexual violence, they may develop *post-traumatic stress disorder (PTSD).* The trauma can be:

1. Directly experienced by the individual
2. Witnessed as happening to another
3. Learning the event happened to a loved one, or
4. Work-related, with the extreme exposure to aversive details of horrific events (e.g., first aid responders repeatedly having to clean up human remains, law enforcement repeatedly exposed to details of sexual abuse against children).

The 4 major symptom clusters for PTSD are

1. Intrusion symptoms (re-experiencing of the event) — For example, sudden memories, dreams, or flashbacks related to the event.
2. Heightened arousal — For example, reckless or self-destructive behavior, as well as sleep disturbances, hypervigilance, startle responses, or aggressiveness.
3. Avoidance — Staying away from places, events, or objects that are reminders of the experience.
4. Negative thoughts and mood or feelings — For example, individuals may be unable to experience positive emotions. They may feel a sense of blame towards themselves or others about the event. They may have markedly diminished interest in activities or an inability to remember major aspects of the event.

The *PTSD Dissociative Subtype* is diagnosed when PTSD is observed with prominent dissociative symptoms. These dissociative symptoms can be either experiences of feeling detached from one's own mind and body, or experiences in which the world seems unreal, dreamlike, or distorted. Some 15-30% of individuals with PTSD have these symptoms. When the symptom last longer than 1 month, the diagnosis of PTSD is given. When the symptoms occur within 4 weeks of the traumatic event and resolve within 4 weeks, the diagnosis given is called *Acute Stress Disorder*.

Adjustment Disorders are diagnosed when behavioral and emotional symptoms emerge within 3 months of a stressor and don't persist for more than 6 months after the stressor has terminated. Individuals who don't meet the criteria for a range of disorders are often diagnosed with an adjustment disorder if the symptoms cause significant impairment and marked distress. The subtypes include *with depressed mood, with anxiety,* or *disturbances in conduct.*

Dissociative Identity Disorder (DID) was previously known as *multiple personality disorder.* It is a controversial diagnosis, where an individual has two or more distinct personality states. The transitions in identity may be self-reported or observed by others. The person also tends to have significant gaps in recall for everyday events and the traumatic events. *Dissociative amnesia* (the individual is distressed due to the inability to recall important facts about herself, usually related to traumatic experience) and *depersonalization/derealization disorder* are related conditions (the individual is distressed due to experiencing himself as unreal [*depersonalization*] or aspects of the world as unreal [*derealization*]).

TREATMENT CONSIDERATIONS

Psychotherapy for Anxiety Disorders

Cognitive behavior therapy (CBT) is often the first-line treatment for anxiety disorders, especially panic disorder. The treatment of Post-traumatic Stress Disorder is described below. Obsessive-Compulsive Disorder most often requires a combination of medication and psychotherapy, specifically CBT with an emphasis on the behavior therapy components of exposure therapy and response prevention. Panic Disorder may require both medication and psychotherapy.

Medications for Anxiety Disorders

- Although benzodiazepines such as *diazepam* (Valium), *lorazepam* (Ativan), *alprazolam* (Xanax) and *clonazepam* (Klonopin) quickly alleviate anxiety in many situations, they are habituating and have marked potential for abuse. In addition, these drugs, especially when used frequently, may impair an individual's capacity to effectively manage his or her anxiety problems in the long term. However, used judiciously as noted above (e.g., only weekly, or less often, in acute panic situations), they may be a very effective adjunctive treatment.

- Serotonin selective reuptake inhibitors (SSRIs), which are classified as anti-depressants, are probably the most effective and safest medications for many anxiety disorders. In fact, the SSRIs have many more FDA indications for anxiety disorders.
- Some serotonin/norepinephrine reuptake inhibitors also have FDA indications for anxiety disorders.
- The tricyclic antidepressant *clomipramine* has potent serotonin reuptake inhibition and may be very effective in OCD.
- *Buspirone* is a serotonergic drug for generalized anxiety that may be very helpful in some patients, particularly those that have not taken benzodiazepines.
- *Hydroxyzine* is an antihistamine that also is useful in some patients.
- Many other drugs are at times used for anxiety "off label," i.e., without an FDA indication, including *propranolol*, *gabapentin*, and *baclofen*. Each of these agents may be effective in certain patients.

The above treatment considerations may vary depending on the following specific diagnoses:

Treatment of Social Anxiety Disorder:

Desensitization therapy (gradually increasing the exposure of the patient to the feared situation) usually successfully treats phobias. Cognitive Behavior Therapy (CBT) using cognitive restructuring and relaxation techniques is also used (for more information see the psychotherapy section). Finally, serotonin selective reuptake inhibitors (SSRIs) in the same doses that are effective for depression are often used as adjunctive therapy. Benzodiazepines have been commonly used but may actually prevent recovery by diminishing the effectiveness of exposure therapy.

Treatment of Panic Disorder:

The psychosocial treatment for panic disorder includes CBT and panic-focused psychodynamic psychotherapy. First-line medications are SSRIs and serotonin-norepinephrine reuptake inhibitors (SNRIs). The judicious use of benzodiazepines with careful monitoring in those who do not have a history of a substance use disorder may also be indicated for prn use (as noted above).

Treatment of Generalized Anxiety Disorder:

Psychotherapy (CBT, psychodynamic or supportive psychotherapy) is the treatment of choice. SSRI's and SNRI's may be helpful in GAD; *buspirone* is also helpful for some patients. Because of the rapid development of tolerance with daily use, benzodiazepines are of little benefit in this condition.

Treatment of Post-traumatic Stress Disorder:

The treatment for PTSD is *psychotherapy*, including *cognitive processing therapy (CPT)*, *prolonged exposure (PE)*, and *eye movement desensitization & reprocessing therapy (EMDR)*. Cognitive therapies aim to alter the meaning and implications of the trauma. Exposure-based therapies involve systematic exposure and desensitization to trauma, while incorporating relaxation techniques. EMDR has been shown to be helpful in desensitizing patients to traumatic memories, thus allowing them to feel significantly less anxious when traumatic memories occur in the future.

Two SSRIs, the antidepressant medications *sertraline* and *paroxetine*, are the only agents approved by the FDA for PTSD and are often helpful in reducing irritability and anxiety. Other SSRIs and SNRIs are also useful for PTSD; their doses are the same as for the treatment of depressive disorders. Antianxiety medications are also occasionally helpful, but the Veterans Administration (VA) National Center for PTSD has determined that benzodiazepines are contraindicated in PTSD as they may actually interfere with recovery.

Prazosin, an alpha adrenergic receptor blocker with FDA approval as an antihypertensive, has been found to be helpful in reducing nightmares. However, a more recent randomized controlled trial found that prazosin was no better than placebo in reducing nightmares in veterans with chronic PTSD.

In more severe cases, antipsychotic medications have been used, though recent studies have questioned their efficacy.

Treatment of Obsessive-Compulsive Disorder:
Effective treatment of obsessive-compulsive disorder usually consists of psychotherapy, behavior modification (focusing on exposure and response prevention), and medication (usually high or even maximum doses of SSRIs (e.g., *fluoxetine* 60-80mg/day, *paroxetine* 40-60mg/day).

Clomipramine is in the chemical class of tricyclic antidepressants, but its FDA approval is only for obsessive-compulsive disorder.

(See Chapter 16, Treatment Modalities, for further discussion of treatment options.)

CHAPTER 8. ALCOHOL AND SUBSTANCE USE DISORDERS

Addiction has been defined by George Koob and Michel Le Moal as a "chronic relapsing disorder characterized by compulsive drug seeking, a loss of control in limiting intake, and the emergence of a negative emotional state when access to the drug is prevented." The addictive process is highly complex. It involves many neural circuits, and the brain undergoes many molecular and neurochemical changes with substance abuse. In addiction, both genes and environment can significantly impact brain functioning and behavior.

In DSM-5, the distinction between substance "abuse" and "dependence" has been replaced with the diagnosis of *"substance use disorder" (SUD)*. Each substance use disorder is then divided into mild, moderate, and severe subtypes. To be diagnosed with substance use disorder, 2 out of 11 criteria must be met. These criteria include:

1. Larger amounts of substance taken than intended
2. Persistent desire to cut down, or control use
3. Great deal of time to obtain, use, or recover
4. Failure to fulfill role obligations
5. Use despite social/interpersonal problems
6. Activities given up or reduced
7. Use in situations where it is physically hazardous
8. Use despite physical/psychological problems
9. Craving or strong desire to use
10. Tolerance: the person needs more and more of the substance to achieve the desired effect.
11. Withdrawal: the person develops a specific set of reversible symptoms after stopping the use of the substance. It is usually opposite to the direct pharmacological effects of a drug.

The tolerance and withdrawal criteria do not apply if the medication is prescribed and adhered to by the patient.

Alcoholism (Alcohol Use Disorder)

Alcohol use is common in American culture, and most people who drink socially do not develop medical or psychological problems. When alcohol is abused, it poses a major public health problem. You may have heard the rumor that alcoholism has replaced syphilis in Osler's famous phrase, "He who knows [this disease] knows medicine."

About 55% of Americans drink alcohol. Approximately 7% are heavy drinkers. This amounts to approximately 10-20 million Americans. A significant number of patients hospitalized in general medical hospitals have alcohol-related problems. Cirrhosis of the liver, a problem frequently associated with serious alcohol use disorders, is the eighth leading cause of death in the USA. In some areas, 50% of homicide victims are legally intoxicated; 20% or more of suicide victims are legally intoxicated; at least 50% of fatal automobile accidents are associated with alcohol abuse.

So-called "accidental deaths" are the fourth leading cause of death overall and the number 1 cause of death in both men and women up to age 34. Many of these "accidental deaths" are caused by burns and carbon monoxide poisoning. Many are alcohol-related. Alcoholism affects all socioeconomic groups, but more men are affected than women.

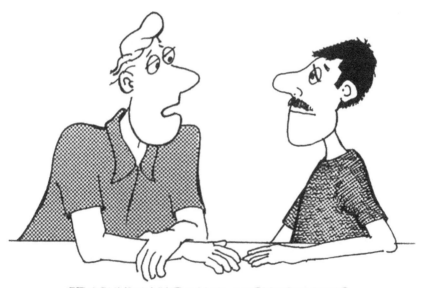

IT SOUNDS LIKE I HAD A TERRIFIC TIME LAST NIGHT...........WHAT DID I DO AFTER I CLIMBED THE FLAGPOLE?

Fig. 8-1. Alcoholism and memory.

Many factors are thought to contribute to alcoholism. Patients with a family history of alcoholism are more likely to develop alcoholism in adult life. Cultural influences are also extremely important. In some cultures, alcohol use is frowned upon but intoxication is implicitly accepted. In other cultures, alcohol use is the norm but intoxication is unacceptable. The availability of alcohol leads to its use. This is obviously an important issue in setting age limits on alcohol use. A history of trauma in individuals with antisocial and borderline personality disorders is associated with an increased risk of developing alcoholism.

Before discussing the treatment of alcohol use disorders, let's run through the myriad complications seen in more severe alcohol use disorders. First are the "medical" complications. Gastrointestinal disease (peptic ulcer, gastritis), liver disease (hepatitis, alcoholic fatty liver, cirrhosis and its attendant problems), pancreatitis, cardiomyopathy, anemia, myopathy, and hypoglycemia are all complications of alcoholism.

The neurologic complications include peripheral neuropathy, dementia, cerebellar degeneration, subdural hematomas, and Wernicke-Korsakoff syndrome. This last problem is a life-threatening illness caused by *thiamine* deficiency that alcoholics may develop. It includes confusion and apathy, ataxia, and abnormal eye movements. If treatment is not instituted (*thiamine* 100mg IM/IV daily for 3 days followed by 100mg PO TID for 2 weeks), this illness progresses to the irreversible Korsakoff's dementia (anterograde amnesia with confabulation—making up facts—and severe memory impairment). Korsakoff's syndrome has a 20% recovery rate.

Alcohol withdrawal syndromes can be life threatening! As a general principle, all sedatives (including alcohol) can cause severe, even deadly, withdrawal problems:

1. Alcohol withdrawal consists of anxiety, psychomotor agitation, sweating, mildly elevated vital signs, tremor, mild confusion, and discomfort. It can start 8-12 hours following the last drink and last up to 48 hours. These withdrawal symptoms are NOT life threatening. Some discomfort may continue for days.
2. Withdrawal seizures develop 12–36 hours following the last drink. Remember that a variety of other problems could cause seizures in an alcoholic, including infection, head trauma, and metabolic problems.
3. Alcoholic hallucinosis can develop 12-24 hours after the last drink and consists of auditory hallucinations in a patient with an otherwise normal mental status examination.
4. *Delirium tremens (DTs)* is a life-threatening alcohol withdrawal state that consists of delirium, often with visual hallucinations. The mortality rate is up to 20%. This syndrome develops later (between 72-96 hours after last drink) and lasts up to 10 days. Admission to a medical unit is usually essential; benzodiazepines and supportive medical management are required.

Treatment of Alcohol Use Disorder

Patients in alcohol withdrawal require medical evaluation and monitoring. Those with mild to moderate alcohol withdrawal and no history of severe alcohol withdrawal, such as seizures or DTs, may be considered for medically monitored outpatient alcohol withdrawal. These patients may be treated with oral thiamine, folic acid, and multivitamins, adequate hydration, and a gradually decreasing dose of a benzodiazepine. This treatment can be monitored with frequent visits to the physician's office. Recent research findings suggest that *gabapentin* may be an alternative medication for detoxification in these patients, and there are published protocols using this agent.

Most patients with moderate or severe alcohol withdrawal require admission to a hospital to safely treat and monitor withdrawal and prevent, if possible, the development of DTs. Initial treatment begins with intravenous thiamine and hydration and is quickly followed by treatment with benzodiazepines, using a symptom-triggered withdrawal protocol incorporating the Clinical Institute Withdrawal Assessment for Alcohol. While no one benzodiazepine is superior, it is helpful to remember that patients with compromised livers should receive a benzodiazepine that is metabolized outside the liver. These include *lorazepam*, which may be the most frequently used agent, as well as *oxazepam* and *temazepam*. Think "outside the liver."

A toxicology screen or blood alcohol level can usually tell whether someone has recently been drinking alcohol, but it does not confirm the number of years that the patient has been drinking. Other tests that the clinician can order to help understand the pattern of use are gamma-glutamyl transferase (GGT) and carbohydrate deficient transferrin (CDT). A ratio of aspartate transaminase (AST) to alanine transaminase (ALT) that is greater than 2:1 is suggestive of alcoholic liver disease. Patients may also have macrocytic anemia with elevated mean corpuscular volume (MCV), which suggests chronic heavy drinking in patients who acknowledge alcohol use.

Alcohol treatment can have several components, including biological treatment (medications), psychological therapy, and social/spiritual interventions. In the acute setting, detox is often needed followed by rehab!

Three FDA-approved medications for alcohol use disorders are *disulfiram*, which inhibits aldehyde dehydrogenase, an enzyme in the metabolism of alcohol (a person who drinks alcohol will then become very nauseous and sick); *naltrexone*, which may reduce alcohol craving; and *acamprosate*, which may also reduce drinking days in patients in recovery. In addition to these agents, *gabapentin* has recently been shown to reduce relapse and heavy drinking in the rehabilitation phase, post-detoxification, but does not have an FDA indication for this purpose.

Treatment for alcoholism can be divided into *withdrawal management* (described above), *rehabilitation*, and *follow-up with support*:

The *rehabilitation* phase of alcoholism treatment is variable in length. This phase of treatment may be accomplished on an inpatient or outpatient basis. When the patient has a previous history of DTs, very poor impulse control (frequent fights, spending binges), a history of seizures, or major underlying psychiatric problems, the treatment should begin inpatient. Education about the physiological and psychological effects of alcohol, including how the patient's alcoholism affects the patient's relatives, employer, etc., is essential. Clinicians should also treat underlying co-occurring psychiatric diagnoses when the patient is free from substance use. Treatment should aim to help the alcoholic find a way to replace alcohol in his or her life. Group therapy, individual therapy, and self-help programs like Alcoholics Anonymous (AA) or SMART Recovery can help in this regard.

The last phase of treatment consists of *support*. Most experts in the field believe that the only reasonable goal for an alcoholic is to completely abstain from drinking. Some experts believe that a subtype of drinkers can work towards controlled drinking. AA, family, friends, business, psychiatrist, or a combination of the above should be used as support. Allowing an alcoholic to become socially isolated may cause relapse.

(See Chapter 16, Treatment Modalities, for further discussion of treatment options.)

Other Substance Use Disorders

We will provide brief clinical descriptions of the effects of a variety of substances that can pose significant health risks to individuals.

Narcotics (Opioids)

Narcotics (heroin, morphine, oxycodone, meperidine, fentanyl, codeine, etc.) produce physical and psychological dependence. They therefore cause a withdrawal syndrome after prolonged abuse. Today, narcotics cause a major public health concern with people from all walks of life getting "hooked" on them. The use of prescription painkillers, as well as heroin, has significantly increased in the last decade. Initially, narcotics are prescribed after surgery or for bona fide conditions that require the use of pain alleviation. Unfortunately, they can also become highly addictive.

Heroin intoxication causes drowsiness, respiratory depression, euphoria, pain relief, nausea, vomiting, and pupil constriction. Excess narcotic use can cause coma and death.

Narcotic withdrawal is similar to a flu-like syndrome that is not life threatening (unless the person has underlying severe medical problems). This withdrawal is extremely uncomfortable, with acute symptoms such as irritability, anxiety, pupil dilation, yawning, and gastrointestinal distress, which can last up to a week. Symptoms that can last significantly longer include intense cravings, depressed mood, muscle aches and pains, insomnia, decreased appetite, and reduced libido.

Sedatives, Hallucinogens, and Marijuana

Sedatives (benzodiazepines and barbiturates) have the potential for psychological and physical addiction. Withdrawal from these drugs, like alcohol (which is also a sedative), can be life-threatening and should usually be initiated in an inpatient unit.

Hallucinogens (e.g., LSD, psilocybin, mescaline, ecstasy) cause perceptual disturbances, including illusions (misperceiving actual sensory stimuli), hallucinations, derealization, and depersonalization. Some people may become very paranoid, depressed, and anxious. It is necessary to treat acute intoxication with a quiet room and "talking down" (lots of reassurance), and sometimes antipsychotic or benzodiazepine medication. These drugs may have anticholinergic properties, too. Anticholinergic drugs may cause dry mouth, constipation, dilated pupils, hyperthermia, tachycardia, and delirium. Many people who used LSD chronically in the 1960s continue to experience flashbacks. Hydration is crucial during overdose of MDMA (ecstasy).

Marijuana use is widespread in America today. Tetrahydrocannabinol (THC) is the psychoactive ingredient and is not always harmless. The acute effects of marijuana include sedation, euphoria, pupillary constriction, and a sense of timelessness. Some people who use marijuana will experience paranoia, and some may even have panic attacks. Rarely, marijuana can induce a transient psychosis lasting several hours to several days after its use. Long-term use can cause decreased sperm count and cause lethargy, chronic bronchitis, or lung cancer. Habitual use may also lead to an "unmotivated" syndrome. *Cannabis withdrawal* is now a bona fide condition in DSM-5; cessation can cause irritability, anxiety, and depression, in addition to somatic complaints.

However, marijuana also has some promising therapeutic effects. It can reduce nausea and vomiting, such as during chemotherapy. It may also have a beneficial effect on glaucoma, although it is effective for only a short time, after which tolerance develops.

Stimulants

Stimulants include cocaine, crack, amphetamines, and crystal meth. Cocaine is an anesthetic that produces euphoria and optimism, making it particularly psychologically appealing. It is also physically addictive. The method of cocaine usage likely correlates with whether an habitual pattern of use develops. Cocaine can be snorted, smoked ("crack"), or used intravenously. Common transient side effects of cocaine are impaired judgment, elevated vital signs (cocaine has sympathomimetic properties), and grandiosity. Uncommon side effects include transient psychosis (lasting as long as several days after use), hyperthermia, seizures, and circulatory collapse.

Amphetamines are used for stimulating and arousing properties. Common side effects include euphoria, anorexia, dry mouth, and elevated vital signs. Less common side effects include motor movements, seizures, and circulatory collapse. Psychiatrists are especially interested in one particular side effect. Some cocaine users develop a transient paranoid psychosis (lasting hours to several weeks) that may be indistinguishable from paranoid schizophrenia. The drug dosage at which this occurs can vary with the individual. Chronic abuse of amphetamines causes tolerance, and withdrawal from amphetamines can cause depression.

Crystal meth has become a major public health problem, particularly on the West Coast of the USA. Individuals can "cook it" in their own kitchens, and this type of stimulant produces a longer-lasting high than cocaine. People develop what is known as "meth mouth and crank bugs" when their teeth become severely decayed and they lose teeth.

Nicotine use continues to be a major public health problem. Smoking causes increased morbidity and mortality, including cardiovascular disease and lung cancer.

Caffeine. In recent years, emergency rooms have seen a significant increase in problems related to consumption of high levels of caffeine (found in energy drinks such as Red Bull), which often occurs in combination with other drugs and alcohol. Caffeine is the most abused substance in the world. Caffeine intoxication and withdrawal are real.

Other Drugs

Various other drugs come in and out of vogue, including *inhalants* (paint and glue sniffing), *anabolic steroids*, and *PCP*. Different synthetic drugs like *bath salts*, *Spice/K2*, *gamma-hydroxybutyric acid (GHB)* are increasing in popularity. Substance misuse is a frequent cause of severe agitation in emergency room patients. With increased access to information over the Internet, people can more easily obtain different synthetic substances for recreational use. Clinicians dealing with such patients must become aware of these new substances and their management.

Always remember to order a urinary toxicology in patients that you suspect might be using drugs. When addressing issues of substance misuse, always approach the patient in a nonjudgmental, caring, and supportive way. Ask open-ended questions and find out what patient's' reasons are for wanting to make a change in their life.

When a person suffers from a co-occurring mental illness and addiction, assessment is key, and it is important for the clinician to take a very detailed history. The clinician needs to know if the psychiatric symptoms are present only in the context of substance use or are present when the person was not using the substance. While in-depth treatment of this population is outside the scope of this book, it is important to remember that recovery includes addressing both the substance issue and any underlying mood, anxiety, and psychotic disorders.

Within the last decade, it has been recognized that "behavioral" addictions, such as gambling, share the same core features as substance addictions. While *Gambling Disorder* now falls under the "Substance Use and Addictive Disorders" section of the DSM-5, other behavioral addictions such as *Internet Use Disorder* and *Hypersexual Disorder* are subsumed under Section III, which is the section of DSM-5 reserved for conditions that require further research. The remainder of the behavioral addictions fall under the obsessive end of the Obsessive-Compulsive and Related Disorders and the impulsive end of the Disruptive, Impulse Control, and Conduct Disorders. Behavioral addictions (i.e., sex, food, tanning, exercise) remain a very controversial topic in psychiatry.

TREATMENT CONSIDERATIONS

Treatment of Other Substance Use Disorders

Drug programs for opioid addicts that provide patients with support, potentially a medication, and a new "culture" (i.e., new peers who do not support drug abuse or antisocial behavior) are effective treatments. The 3 medications used in the treatment of opioid use disorders are *methadone* (full opiate receptor agonist), *buprenorphine* (partial opiate agonist), and *naltrexone* (opioid antagonist). People who inject heroin with shared needles are at a heightened risk of contracting Hepatitis C or HIV.

Management of withdrawal and rehabilitation for patients with sedative abuse and dependence (primarily patients who abuse benzodiazepines) is the same as for those addicted to alcohol.

Habitual stimulant abuse (whether cocaine or amphetamines) is difficult to treat. Successful programs likely have to be coercive to succeed (e.g., threaten to turn the user in to his employer if traces of cocaine are present in the user's body). In some cocaine users, drug usage takes priority over family and job. Therefore, family counseling may help a family cope with its affected member. Sentences to treatment within the correctional system is a fact of life for some addicted to these drugs.

Psychoeducation with all nicotine users is essential. There are various nicotine replacement therapies available on the market (including patches, gum, and lozenges), in addition to bupropion and varenicline. Patients should also be referred to psychosocial treatments, including CBT. Nicotine withdrawal is extremely unpleasant and usually includes intense cravings, depressed mood, insomnia, irritability, weight gain, and increased appetite.

(See Chapter 16, Treatment Modalities, for further discussion of treatment options.)

CHAPTER 9.   THE SLEEPLESS PATIENT

Sleep is a vital human behavior. Impaired sleep can result in negative medical, psychiatric, and psychosocial consequences. While sleep disorders are rarely life threatening (except sleep apnea), they can cause enough distress to warrant careful workup and treatment.

A word or 2 about sleep physiology is in order. Sleep normally progresses through 4 stages. After stage 3, REM (rapid eye movement sleep, when people dream) occurs. The deep stages of sleep (N3) predominate early in the night, while REM sleep is more common later in the night. Passing from stage 1 to REM sleep takes about 90 minutes. Then the sleeper goes back to stage 1, then back to REM, and so on.

NREM Stage 1 → The stage between sleep and wakefulness (alpha activity predominated)
NREM Stage 2 → (theta activity)
NREM Stage 3 → Slow-wave sleep (beginning of delta activity)
REM

As people age, there is a significant increase in N1-N2 (light sleep) and decrease in N3 (deep sleep). The amount of time spent in REM (deep sleep) also decreases. Older people also often take longer to fall asleep, may have more nighttime awakenings, and may have decreased perceived restfulness.

Ten disorders fall under sleep-wake disorders in DSM-5. These include *insomnia disorder*, *hypersomnolence disorder*, *narcolepsy*, *breathing-related sleep disorders*, *circadian rhythm sleep disorders*, *non-REM (NREM) sleep arousal disorders*, *nightmare disorder*, *REM sleep behavior disorder*, *restless legs syndrome*, and *substance-or medication-induced sleep disorder*.

Insomnia Disorder

Insomnia Disorder is diagnosed when a patient has difficulty initiating or maintaining sleep or complains that he or she sleeps but does not feel rested. Below is a list of conditions or factors that may cause insomnia. Remember that for Insomnia Disorder, underlying mental/substance/medical conditions do not adequately explain the insomnia. Treatment for Insomnia Disorder may include psychoeducation about sleep hygiene, CBT, and sedative hypnotic agents. To organize your thinking about insomnia, just remember **DEEP**. *Drugs, Environment, Emotions,* and *Physical* (medical) problems can cause insomnia.

D: *Drugs.* Any drug with diuretic action can cause trouble sleeping because the patient has to get up to void. Beta-blockers (like *propranolol*), *digitalis*, antidepressants, *pentazocine*, and *baclofen* can cause nightmares. Obviously, a *Drug* history is important in the workup of insomnia.

E: *Environment.* A surprising number of cases of insomnia are caused by *Environmental* problems (e.g., noise, other stress). A snoring spouse or noisy home may make sleeping difficult (**Fig. 9-1**). Irregular work shifts or sleeping in a strange bed can also cause sleep disruption. Worries about an exam or another upcoming stressor may also transiently disrupt sleep.

E: *Emotional.* While worrying may cause a fitful night's rest, moderate or severe psychiatric illnesses can cause profound sleep disruption. Mild depression causes patients to have trouble falling asleep, and severe depression also results in early morning awakening. Mania causes so much agitation that sleeping is almost impossible. More severe anxiety consistently affects sleep patterns. Schizophrenia probably does not specifically affect sleep, but it does cause agitation and anxiety, which affect sleep. Delirium usually causes gross disruption of the sleep-wake cycle. Paranoid people may not be willing to let their guard down for long enough to sleep. The above disorders are discussed at length in their respective chapters.

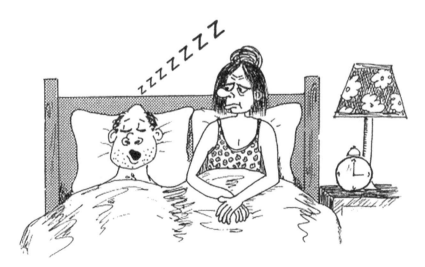

Fig. 9-1.   The Environment is noisy.

P: *Physical problems.* Anyone in *Pain* is going to have trouble falling asleep. It is harder to stay distracted when trying to fall asleep at night, than it is during the day, and distraction keeps one's mind off pain. The antidepressant *amitriptyline* often helps with sleep disturbance caused by chronic pain and may decrease pain as well.

Likewise, medical illnesses, particularly those requiring hospitalization, can cause sleeping problems. Certain medical conditions actually strike at night or during sleep (paroxysmal nocturnal dyspnea secondary to heart failure, nocturnal angina). Short-term usage of hypnotic drugs may be indicated, as long as the drugs don't aggravate the underlying condition.

The differential diagnosis of sleep trouble is relatively simple. A sleep lab can help firm up a diagnosis by running a sleeping EEG on your patient. You can help a lot of people if you can get them to sleep. Just remember **DEEP**!

Hypersomnolence Disorder is present when an individual self-reports excessive sleepiness throughout the day; even after more than 9 hours of sleep that person still feels tired.

Narcolepsy, on the other hand, consists of *cataplexy* (sudden loss of motor tone when the patient experiences a strong emotion), daytime drowsiness, *sleep paralysis* (upon awakening, the patient is transiently paralyzed), and hypnogogic hallucinations (hallucinations experienced on falling asleep). Narcolepsy is associated with hypocretin deficiency. Sleeping EEGs (electroencephalograms) demonstrate that REM sleep, in narcolepsy, occurs at sleep onset rather than its usual appearance after stages 1 to 4. Treatment consists of psychostimulants. Certain antidepressants (TCAs and SSRIs) are also known to decrease REM interruption.

Breathing-Related Sleep Disorders are split into *Obstructive Sleep Apnea Hypopnea* (airway obstruction during sleep), *Central Sleep Apnea* (caused by variability in respiratory effort), and *Sleep-Related Hypoventilation* (often comorbid with neurological conditions, medication, or substances). *Sleep apnea* is a condition of respiratory pause during sleep that leads to multiple short arousals, often to hypoxia and hypercarbia (increased pCO_2), and to the sense of having a poor night's sleep. Central Sleep Apnea is presumed secondary to a problem in the respiratory center of the brain. Obstructive Sleep Apnea Hypopnea is thought to be caused by anatomical closure of the upper airways, especially the pharynx, during sleep. Occasionally, obesity or hypothyroidism are associated with sleep apnea.

Severe complications can arise with these illnesses. Hypoxia can cause cardiac arrhythmias and cor pulmonale. Daytime drowsiness can be severe. Treatment may consist of weight loss (which presumably reduces fat tissue in the pharynx), nighttime monitoring, or the daytime use of stimulants. Central nervous system depressants like alcohol and sedative-hypnotics should NOT be used because they aggravate the problem.

Circadian Rhythm Sleep-Wake Disorder results from a mismatch between endogenous circadian rhythm and the sleep-wake schedule required by the person's environment. Various subtypes exist; *delayed phase type* ("night owls"), *advanced phase type* (people who go to bed very, very early), and *shift-work type* are the most common.

Parasomnias

Parasomnias are sleep disorders resulting in abnormal behaviors in the deep stages of sleep (stage 3 and REM). The parasomnias include:

- *Sleepwalking*: Contrary to what we see in popular cartoons in which a character gracefully and aimlessly walks a tightrope while sleepwalking, this disorder (*somnambulism*) may occasionally be dangerous. Patients can trip, fall, and hurt themselves. Patients who sleepwalk should have their room secured so that there is nothing dangerous to walk into. Otherwise, this condition is fairly benign. It, too, can be triggered by daytime stress.
- *Sleep Terrors*: Sleep terror is an awakening in the deep stages of sleep accompanied by loud screaming and frenetic behavior. The scream may be so blood curdling as to strike panic in the rest of the family, but the condition is normally very benign and self-limited. Occasionally, sleep terrors are precipitated by daytime stress. For that reason, a cursory history should be taken to ensure that the patient is not being abused, experiencing inordinate stress, or having other difficulties. Sleep terrors can be distinguished from nightmares fairly easily.
- *Nightmare Disorder*: Nightmares are associated with dreams. They occur later in the sleep cycle during REM sleep, usually in individuals who can be wakened without great difficulty.
- *Rapid Eye Movement Sleep Behavior Disorder*: This disorder is seen in elderly people whose violent motor activity causes injury to the self or to bed partners. Usually the muscles are not moving during REM sleep.
- *Restless Legs Syndrome*: This syndrome creates an urge to move one's legs in response to uncomfortable sensations in the legs.

Again, just remember **DEEP,** and you can help people with sleep problems.

TREATMENT CONSIDERATIONS

Treatment of Insomnia Disorder

Psychotherapy

Cognitive behavior therapy for insomnia (CBT-I) has been shown to be as effective as medications in some studies.

Medications

Sedative hypnotic agents have been used for many years for insomnia. Currently the GABA agonists *zolpidem* and *eszopiclone* are the most widely used. Benzodiazepines that specifically have FDA indications for sleep include *temazepam*, *flurazepam, triazolam,* and others. All of these drugs may lead to tolerance and rebound insomnia and are most prudently used if limited to only a few weeks.

Other drugs or drug classes that are sedating include antihistamines (especially *diphenhydramine, doxylamine,* and *hydroxyzine*) and some antidepressants, including *trazodone* and *mirtazapine.* Older tricyclic antidepressants are used as well, especially *amitriptyline* and *doxepin.*

In addition to the above agents, *melatonin,* a hormone produced by the pineal gland in the brain and related to the natural sleep cycle, is available as a non-prescription sleep aid. It has been shown to be helpful for sleep in some studies; a melatonin receptor agonist, *ramelteon,* is available as a prescription drug.

(See Chapter 16, Treatment Modalities, for further discussion of treatment options.)

CHAPTER 10.   EATING DISORDERS

Anorexia Nervosa and Bulimia Nervosa

Although we value humor, there is nothing funny about a person suffering from *anorexia nervosa (AN)* or *bulimia nervosa (BN)*. These illnesses, particularly anorexia nervosa, can be *devastating*. They affect individuals of all races, ethnicities, and socioeconomic backgrounds, although there is an approximately 10:1 female to male ratio (the number of males has begun to increase). Psychological anguish experienced by such children and adults is severe; the frustration experienced by families is often extreme. Diagnosing an eating disorder can be difficult because many suffer in silence, do not seek treatment, and keep the behavior very private. The other main types of eating disorders that this chapter will cover are *Binge Eating Disorder (BED)* and *Avoidant Restrictive Food Intake Disorder (ARFD)*. Patients who do not fall neatly into the diagnostic categories of AN, BN, BED, or ARFD receive the diagnosis of Eating Disorder NOS (Not Otherwise Specified). EDNOS is the #1 diagnosed eating disorder in clinical settings.

To make this subject more palatable, we've begun by arranging the key diagnostic findings for AN into an acronym, **LOW FOOD.** The diagnostic findings in anorexia nervosa are:

L: *Loss*
O: *Of*
W: *Weight:* There is a weight loss with a BMI < 18.5 or, for moderate to severe cases, < 17.
F: *Fear*
Of
O: *Obesity:* These individuals are terrified about being fat.
D: *Distortion* of body image manifested by the belief of these individuals that they are overweight despite actually being emaciated (**Fig. 10-1**).

Refusal to eat occurs despite family and medical intervention. Miscellaneous symptoms, most of which are secondary to weight loss include anemia, amenorrhea, lanugo hair growth, bradycardia, QT abnormalities, osteoporosis, seizures or delirium, vomiting and purging, and laxative abuse. There are 2 subgroups of

AN: *restricting type* with no purging or binge eating; and *binge eating-purging type* with low weight plus self-induced vomiting or misuse of laxatives, diuretics, or enemas.

Please look for **LOW FOOD** in anyone who has lost weight. Remember, not every thin child has anorexia nervosa. A variety of medical problems can mimic this psychiatric condition and should not be overlooked. We'll have more to say about the differential diagnosis later.

The incidence of anorexia nervosa is increasing, probably due to social and cultural factors. Thin is beautiful in the U.S.A. One in 200 girls at puberty is now thought to have anorexia nervosa. The disorder is much more common in girls than in boys, and it occurs more commonly in Jewish and Italian families. Middle- and upper-income families are at greater risk for having a child with this disease than are lower socioeconomic status families. The most common age of onset is the teenage years. The illness may be preceded by a period of mild obesity and mild dieting. There is also an association of anorexia nervosa with Turner's syndrome and with above-average intelligence.

No one knows the cause of this disease. Theories about the development of the disorder can be divided into 3 categories:

- The traditional psychoanalytic model assumes that anorexic patients have a deep fear of sexuality and of impregnation. These fears are accompanied by the fantasy that impregnation occurs via the oral route. That's why these patients stop eating, because they don't want to get pregnant! Although this theory is hard to stomach, it does make sense for some of these patients.
- The second, more palatable theory, is one of endocrinologic dysfunction. There are endocrine abnormalities in anorexia nervosa (including increased vasopressin levels and alterations in thyroid function). These may reflect some underlying endocrinological etiology. Girls who develop amenorrhea often do so prior to any significant weight loss. This also suggests that an endocrine imbalance causes this disorder.
- A third theory for the etiology of this condition could be termed an interactional model. Early in childhood there are interactions between parent and child that could lead to a child refusing to eat at an older age. For example, an impatient mother could habitually rush her daughter through meals. This pressure could make it difficult for the girl to enjoy eating. She probably would develop a wish to control her own eating pace. At an older age she might actually refuse to eat.

By now, you are becoming familiar with the diseases in the psychiatric differential diagnosis for anorexia nervosa. Obviously, schizophrenic patients could be delusional about food. They might think that they were being poisoned, and would understandably stop eating. The resulting weight loss could be misperceived as anorexia nervosa. Remember to look for **LOW FOOD.**

Bulimia nervosa (BN) involves recurrent episodes of binge eating followed by some form of purging (including vomiting or increased exercise to atone for overeating) in patients who otherwise maintain their weight. To meet the criteria for

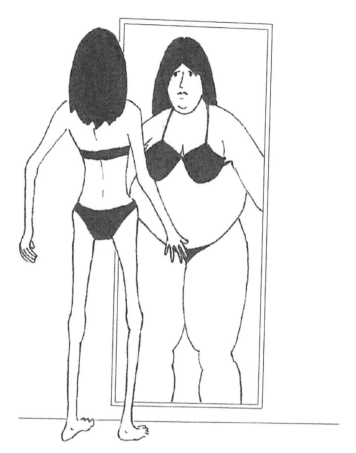

Fig. 10-1.   Anorexia nervosa.

BN, both binge eating and purging must occur at least once a week for 3 months. An important aspect of bulimia is that gross overeating is followed by shame and guilt. Preoccupation with body image is a key aspect of these patients as well. It is important to distinguish depressed patients from patients with eating disorders. Depressed patients often lose weight. too. They usually describe feeling depressed, and report other vegetative signs of depression (remember **ABSTRACT**), and even suicidal ideation. They also don't suffer from **LOW FOOD**.

Patients who suffer from BN often have other psychiatric comorbidities, including mood or anxiety disorders, substance use disorders, or borderline personality disorder (see Chapter 15). These patients tend to have problems with impulsivity in multiple spheres of life and, unlike those with AN, tend to be of average or slightly above or below average weight. BN patients can suffer from electrolyte abnormalities and cardiac arrhythmias similar to AN patients. Repeatedly inducing vomiting can lead to stomach and esophageal tears, and these patients may have menstrual irregularities, nutritional deficiencies, and many other medical problems.

On the medical side of the differential diagnosis are a variety of conditions that should be considered. *Addison's disease* can present with weight loss, anorexia, and vomiting; electrolyte abnormalities should indicate the diagnosis. *Hypothyroidism* may present with cold intolerance, constipation, bradycardia, and skin changes that are similar to those seen in anorexia nervosa. However, hypothyroid patients are often overweight and should have other physical stigmata of this disorder. Other chronic illnesses can cause progressive weight loss, but these should be readily discernible (i.e., inflammatory diseases, chronic infection, and malignancy). Any disorder that causes *panhypopituitarism* could initially mimic anorexia nervosa. The *superior mesenteric artery syndrome* sometimes causes vomiting and anorexia. The vomiting usually occurs when the patient is lying down, though. *Diabetes insipidus (D.I.)* causes excess fluid intake, but behavior and attitudes related to solid food are usually normal. Recent research shows that some schizophrenic patients have D.I. Any patient with D.I. should have a medical workup and mental status examination!

Psychiatric patients with **LOW FOOD** can get into medical difficulty. About 5-15% of anorexic patients die, usually of fluid and electrolyte difficulties. Always check the electrolytes, vital signs, EKG, and mental status of your patient. Why check the mental status when you already have **LOW FOOD**? A small percentage of these patients have recurrent suicidal ideation.

The prognosis is guarded in anorexia nervosa, with many patients never fully recovering from their obsessional concern with weight. Some patients may go on to develop full-blown affective disorders (depression); a few make a full recovery.

Other disorders in this area new in DSM-5 are *Binge Eating Disorder* (binges similar to BN, a feeling of lack of control over eating, but without purging behaviors) and *Avoidant/Restrictive Food Intake Disorder* (marked restriction of food intake, which often leads to physiological and/or psychosocial problems). Eating Disorder NOS continues as in DSM-IV.

Puzzler: Before moving to the next section, we pose a puzzler. Why do so many anorexia nervosa girls appear orange? Is it some odd liver failure syndrome that accompanies starvation?

Obesity

While anorexia nervosa patients may both gain and lose weight, another class of patients gains and never loses — obese patients. This may be one of the least understood of all medical conditions. Certainly the cure rate for severe obesity (100% heavier than ideal weight) is low.

A reasonable approach to understanding and working up obesity is to use a differential diagnosis. First, obesity can be caused by medical problems. Probably, fewer than 5% of obese patients have an underlying medical condition. It doesn't hurt to consider *hypothyroidism, Cushing's disease, Prader-Willi Syndrome* (hypothalamic dysfunction), and side effects of antidepressant and antipsychotic medications and lithium as possible etiologic conditions.

Having ruled these out, move onto the secondary obesity syndromes; i.e., those that are secondary to an underlying psychiatric condition. Obsessional eaters, depressives, anxious people, and even schizophrenics can suffer from obesity because of their underlying condition. The treatment here should be aimed at the underlying problem.

Last, not least, but least understood are the primary obesity syndromes. We list a few hypotheses for why some people become obese:

1. Some patients, fearful of "looking good," choose (unconsciously or consciously) to stay obese so they won't have to deal with intimate relationships or sexuality.
2. Some obese people learn to deal with their frustration or anxiety (beginning at an early age) by eating. They substitute oral gratification for other kinds of gratification.
3. An undiscovered problem with sense of satiety could exist.
4. The set point for eating and weight gain could be set too high in some people, implying that we all tend to stay at approximately the same weight unless this set point changes.

One thing is certain. Psychiatrists don't have much luck using conventional treatments with these people. A psychiatric evaluation may be indicated to rule out other psychiatric conditions, but psychotherapy doesn't usually help. Amphetamines have anorexic properties but aren't safe to use for obesity. Increased risk of medical complications (coronary artery disease, hypertension) is true, especially for the severely obese, but doesn't usually affect the patient's behavior, either.

Psychiatrists are relying more on behavior modification (reinforcing weight loss), nutritional counseling, and their other medical colleagues! In severe obesity, the only effective treatment may be surgery (gastric bypass or related procedures) or supervised caloric restriction.

In moderate obesity (20% heavier than ideal weight), calorie restriction and behavioral modification to encourage weight loss are probably most effective. In mild obesity, no treatment or moderate exercise and calorie restriction may be indicated. Not all obese patients want treatment, and obesity is not synonymous with psychopathology.

Pica is a condition in which people eat non-food substance items (paint chips, dirt, wood, etc.). Iron deficiency can cause pica; many children eat unusual items accidentally or out of curiosity. Although the presence of pica can imply that a child is not being adequately cared for, the side effects of eating odd items are more serious. Lead-based paint chips can cause lead poisoning. Any child with pica should have his or her home environment carefully checked.

And, the answer to the puzzler about orange appearance! No, it's not liver failure. It's *hypercarotenemia*, caused by the ingestion of too many carrots and raw vegetables.

TREATMENT CONSIDERATIONS

Treatment of Anorexia Nervosa

After you have ascertained that your patient with Anorexia Nervosa (AN) is medically stable, the treatment commences. Often an inpatient psychiatric facility will be required to prevent the patient from continuing to diet. Certainly, there is no problem with an outpatient trial of psychotherapy if the patient is not in medical difficulty. You should be aware of things that anorexia nervosa patients do to themselves. A small percentage of them abuse laxatives; a greater percentage self-induce vomiting. Most of these patients distort the amount they are actually eating. This is not done from real maliciousness, but because they are desperate not to gain weight. So, when your anorexia nervosa patient appears at the nurse's desk in the morning with a big smile on her face, two pounds heavier than she was the day before, be suspicious! She may have put metal in her pockets, ingested 3 gallons of water, or put batteries in her shoes. Of course, you may be doing such a superb job, that she has actually gained weight, too. She probably wouldn't be smiling in that instance.

The treatment of these girls should consist of behavioral modification to reinforce *weight gain,* and some combination of individual and family psychotherapy. Family therapy, by a therapist with experience in treating eating disorders, is particularly effective for teens and family members, especially those living in the same household. When a patient's weight drops to a critical point, she should be forced to eat. If she refuses, a nasogastric tube or intravenous hyperalimentation becomes mandatory. It is usually possible to prevent a patient with anorexia nervosa from dying from complications of the disease. A variety of interventions can be made to prevent starvation. There are no FDA approved medications for AN, but medications may be used to treat any comorbid psychiatric disorders.

Treatment of Bulimia Nervosa

Treatment for Bulimia Nervosa (BN) may involve treating electrolyte and acid/base abnormalities. Psychotherapy is crucial, and cognitive behavior therapy (CBT) has been shown to be very effective, especially in conjunction with serotonin reuptake inhibitors (SSRIs). Interpersonal therapy, dialectical behavior therapy (DBT - see Chapter 16), and psychodynamic therapy (see Chapter 16) can also be effective. Encouraging patients to join self-help groups and peer support networks can also help in recovery.

Fluoxetine (Prozac), the first SSRI available in the US, is FDA approved for BN and has been shown to decrease frequency of binges and vomiting. *Bupropion* is contraindicated because it can lower the seizure threshold!

(See Chapter 16, Treatment Modalities, for further discussion of treatment options.)

CHAPTER 11.   PAIN

The differential diagnosis of pain includes a wide variety of psychiatric and physical ailments. The complaint of pain is valid no matter what the underlying diagnosis, and effective pain management is a moral imperative. Remember this and you'll be off to a good start with patients who complain of pain. Eventually you'll form the kind of relationship with them that will alleviate the pain. That's right! When patients believe they are being well cared for, 'they'll feel less pain. This is true whatever the cause of the pain.

Before discussing the differential diagnosis of pain, we would like to say a few words about placebo treatments. Placebos were sometimes used as a way of "proving" that the patient is not in pain. Such misuse of placebos is considered unethical today. A patient's response to a placebo only indicates that the patient is a placebo responder, but does not mean that the patient has no pain. Most likely there are physiological mechanisms that are triggered in response to the suggestion that something will relieve pain. These underlying physiological mechanisms actually do result in pain relief and likely involve endorphin-mediated pain relief. Endorphins are endogenous opioids. In other words, it's great to be a placebo responder! Again, the power of suggestion and a relationship of trust are critical to good patient management.

A complaint of pain, with no identifiable physical reason for the patient to have pain, should lead clinicians to explore the psychiatric differential diagnosis. The remainder of this chapter will discuss this diagnostic category and give you clues and advice on managing such problems. This information is summarized below in **Figure 11-1**.

Pain in Depression

Why does a discussion of depression appear in a chapter on pain? Surprisingly, depression may be the most common cause of pain. Pain can function as a depressive equivalent — a ticket of admission — to the physician's office. Lower back pain, headaches, vague chest pains, and aching extremities may all be presenting complaints for depression.

	Psychological Findings	Affective State	Pain Distribution
Depression	vegetative signs, hopeless, helpless	depressed	lower back pain typical
Somatic Symptom Disorder	strong need to be cared for	anxious	internal organ or varying complaints
Malingering	history of trouble with law, or substance abuse	neutral or angry	story inconsistencies
Factitious Disorder	needs to fool doctors	anxious and demanding	abdominal pain
Conversion (Functional Neurological Symptom Disorder)	the symptom symbolizes something	indifferent or anxious	loss of neurologic functioning often does not follow anatomical pathways

Fig. 11-1.   Pain in psychiatric conditions.

The diagnosis of depression is covered in depth in Chapter 3. Remember, even when patients complain of something other than a depressed mood, it is often possible to diagnose the depressed mood. Simply ask the patient how he or she is feeling and look for other signs of depression. Does the patient appear sad or apathetic? Look for the vegetative signs of depression (anorexia, constipation, sleep disturbance, weight loss, decreased libido). If you suspect depression, a trial of psychotherapy or antidepressants is indicated.

Somatic Symptom Disorder and Illness Anxiety Disorder

Hypochondriasis has been eliminated as a disorder from DSM-5, in part because the name was perceived as pejorative and not conducive to building a good therapeutic relationship. Hypochondriacs believe they have a serious medical illness despite medical assurance to the contrary. Hypochondriacs frequent clinics and private offices in search of someone who will take care of them. Their wish is often frustrated, because many doctors pat such patients on the back, tell them that nothing is wrong, and send them out. If this happens, the patient goes to another doctor's office. The law of averages states that you will occasionally obtain a prescription from a doctor, no matter what your complaint. Consequently, these patients wind up with a list of prescriptions that reads like a hospital formulary.

In DSM-5, individuals with high health anxiety without somatic symptoms receive a diagnosis of *Illness Anxiety Disorder* (unless health anxiety is better explained by a primary anxiety disorder, such as *Generalized Anxiety Disorder).*

If the individual has high health anxiety plus significant somatic complaints, a diagnosis of *Somatic Symptom Disorder* is made.

This type of patient frequently arouses *countertransference* feelings in doctors. Countertransference refers to various feelings doctors have for their patients. Of course, it's important to understand the source of these feelings, often irrational, rather than act on them.

The best way to manage patients with either Illness Anxiety Disorder or Somatic Symptom Disorder is to treat them with understanding care. In other words, take their complaints seriously, listen carefully to their history, tell them that you are worried about them, and see them regularly, albeit briefly. You don't have to give them any medications (unless something is warranted); you also don't have to be a psychiatrist to treat these patients. It's surprising how helpful you can be by showing your concern for your patients. Inevitably, patients with these disorders occasionally develop a "real" illness, too. That's all the more reason for taking their complaints seriously.

Conversion Disorder (Functional Neurological Symptom Disorder)

Conversion Disorder usually refers to a loss of voluntary nervous function without any identifiable physical pathology. Pain without any underlying neurologic problem can also be a conversion disorder. Conversion disorders are uncommon these days. The classical hemipareses, fainting episodes, and hysterical (conversion) seizures of yesteryear just aren't seen as much in the 2000's. Instead, conversion symptoms are more subtle. Vague pain, transient visual disturbances, or transient motor weakness can be conversion symptoms.

From a psychodynamic perspective, the conversion symptom symbolizes the patient's wish to do something and the defense against that wish. For example, a concert pianist could develop numbness and tingling in his fingers for conversion reasons. He can't play the piano because of his symptoms, which functions as a defense against the wish to play piano or be famous.

The differential diagnosis for conversion disorder is extremely important. More than 20% of those diagnosed as having a conversion disorder are found subsequently to have true organic pathology. The psychiatrist and neurologist must be humble when they can't find a reason for the patient's initial loss of motor or sensory functioning. Aside from conversion disorder and the other psychiatric conditions that can cause pain, several neurologic disorders can present like a conversion disorder. Multiple sclerosis often presents with vague neurologic symptoms. The diagnosis of M.S. is based on the development of multiple CNS lesions over a period of time. *Acute intermittent porphyria*, *Wilson's disease* (altered copper metabolism), and small infarcts also may cause symptoms that appear to be conversions, but these are obviously organic problems.

Corroborating psychological data can help lead you to the diagnosis of a conversion disorder. First, conversion patients may appear mildly indifferent to the loss of some significant motor or sensory functioning. This classical "belle indifference" functions like denial, though, so do not place too much importance on this symptom.

If a patient has had previous somatic complaints or conversion symptoms, it's more likely that the current loss is for conversion reasons. If a family member has had a similar neurologic loss, your patient most likely has a conversion symptom, and is identifying with his relative's symptoms. Patients who are the youngest sibling are more prone to have conversion symptoms. A loss of motor or sensory functioning that follows an immediate psychological stressor is more often due to a conversion disorder than a general medical problem.

Unfortunately, conversion disorders can coexist with neurologic conditions. Patients with multiple sclerosis, true seizures, and head trauma seem to be at higher risk for developing conversion symptoms. This obviously adds to the confusion.

Malingering

Malingering is the one exception to the rule to take a patient's complaint of pain seriously. Some patients will come to your office or hospital, complaining of pain, in order to get narcotics or a hospital bed to sleep in. In other words, they aren't actually in pain. They are consciously trying to persuade you to give them something. While some malingerers are drug abusers, many are impoverished patients who have nowhere to spend the night. Although you don't take their complaint of pain seriously, you can still treat them empathically (and also emphatically!).

A diagnosis of malingering should be suspected when the patient does not have any psychological concomitants of the other pain conditions. If the patient has a history of drug abuse, malingering should be suspected. A patient who has been in trouble with the law isn't likely to have many qualms about being dishonest with you, either.

Treat such patients firmly but compassionately. Occasionally, referral to a social service agency will be helpful (to help the patient find a bed for the night, etc.). Often, though, these patients will leave the hospital when they are denied drugs or a hospital bed. Sometimes, these patients are dangerous. If you suspect that the patient you are seeing might try to hurt you, call for help in the form of guards or orderlies. If you have access to a psychiatrist, he or she may be able to help you diagnose malingering and make an appropriate disposition.

Factitious Disorder

Patients with *Factitious Disorder* (formerly known as *Munchausen Syndrome*) consciously want to fool their doctor, but they don't know *why*. These are patients who show up in the emergency room with "gridiron" abdomens and with histories of multiple prior surgeries with nothing ever discovered. Their symptoms and complaints are convincing. Suspect this diagnosis if a patient has a history of multiple surgeries with no reasons (i.e., tumor, disease); if the patient has received medical treatment in many different cities; if the patient is a transient and doesn't have much in the way of family support. Generally, there is no history of drug abuse or other obvious psychopathology. The best management for this condition is psychiatric consultation.

Factitious Disorder by proxy is a type of child abuse whereby a parent induces an illness in his or her child in order to fool the doctor. Examples include injecting toxins into a child or giving a child medicine to make him sick. Invariably the parent is medically trained.

TREATMENT CONSIDERATIONS

Treatment of Pain

The treatment of pain should follow several principles. To reiterate, proving that a patient is a placebo responder does not prove that the patient is pain-free. Secondly, when a patient has acute pathology (e.g., status post abdominal surgery), there is no harm in giving good pain relief with narcotics. Withholding needed pain meds can obviously produce demanding, drug-seeking behavior which, when finally reinforced by the provision of medication, can become a major source of conflict for staff and patient. While providing adequate pain relief is essential, providing time-limited opioid prescriptions with planned discontinuation is critical following acute care as opioid use in the US has reached epidemic proportions, and responsible use is of the utmost importance. Opioids may be essential to ease suffering at the end of life, especially in patients with cancer or other progressively debilitating and fatal disorders. A major dilemma is the effective treatment of chronic non-cancer pain. Effective pain management programs (usually incorporating cognitive behavior therapy in conjunction with other physical therapy and non-opioid pain medications such as acetaminophen, gabapentin, NSAIDs, SNRIs) may be very helpful, depending on the type and source of the pain.

When patients are distracted by a good television show or family visit, they will subjectively experience less pain. Obviously, keeping patients involved in activities is one way to obtain non-narcotic pain control. In the unlikely event that a patient does develop a physiological dependence on narcotics, the withdrawal syndrome for narcotics is generally not life threatening. Narcotics withdrawal is similar to a flu-like condition and poses few medical problems in its management.

Treatment of Conversion Disorder

The treatment of a conversion symptom starts with an honest discussion with a patient. Statements such as, "I'm sorry we don't have an answer, but we think both the psychiatrist and the neurologist should follow you" keep the patient involved in both neurologic and psychiatric care. Hopefully, later the diagnosis will become more obvious. Ultimately, the psychiatric treatment of such patients tries to uncover the symbolism behind the loss of functioning. When a medical student is allowed to discuss how much he wants to slug his resident, his right arm's paralysis may improve. The longer the conversion symptom lasts, the worse the prognosis. Consequently, a patient with a conversion symptom of 3 years duration is less likely to benefit from psychiatric treatment.

CHAPTER 12. MEDICAL PROBLEMS PRESENTING AS PSYCHIATRIC SYNDROMES

Most patients with psychological complaints should have a careful history and physical examination. The history should look for details of medication usage; age of onset of the mental changes; length, type and duration of the mental status changes; and quality of physical complaints. The physical evaluation should include a routine physical examination and a careful neurologic examination. The latter is most likely to reveal helpful information in a patient with an abnormal mental state.

A variety of disorders can cause delirium or dementia (see Chapter 6). This chapter will describe conditions that affect the central nervous system. However, the focus will be on diseases that parade as psychiatric syndromes. It will be your job to rain on the parade of these dysfunctions (**Fig. 12-1**).

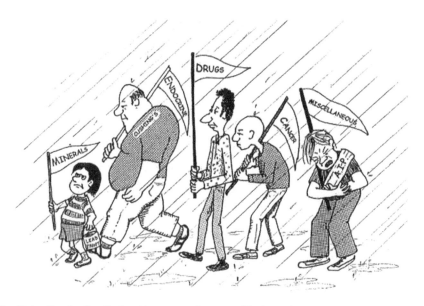

Fig. 12-1. Parade of medical problems presenting as psychiatric syndromes.

A mnemonic to help you categorize these conditions is **MED'CL.** Unfortunately, there will be some hard work in learning the manifestations of these disorders.

M: *Metal poisoning*
E: *Endocrine disorders*
D: *Drug effects*
C: *Cancer*
L: *Lots of others*

M: Metal Poisoning

Lead intoxication can cause intellectual impairment that may progress to delirium and coma. With chronic exposure to lead, the intellectual deficits can be subtle. In massive or acute intoxication, delirium and coma almost always occur.

Lead intoxication should be suspected in a child who behaves abnormally, especially if the child lives in an old house where lead-based paint has been used. Children are more vulnerable than adults to CNS effects. They may become hyperactive, aggressive, or irritable after lead exposure.

In adults, the symptoms of lead poisoning are abdominal pain, neuropathy and anemia. When poisoning is severe, it may present with neurologic changes (dizziness, ataxia, seizures), lead lines (especially in children, at gingival margins), basophilic stippling in the red blood cells, and optic atrophy.

The treatment consists of supportive measures and chelation treatment to help the patient excrete the lead. Early intervention may not prevent permanent CNS damage, so the best treatment is preventative (e.g., use of unleaded paint, gasoline).

Mercury poisoning causes personality changes, characteristically increased timidity, withdrawal, easy embarrassment, and irritability. The physical changes associated with mercury poisoning include stomatitis, possible kidney and lung disease, insomnia, fatigue and even hallucinations. The neurologic changes are ataxia and tremor. The treatment is a chelator such as penicillamine to help the patient excrete the metal. The personality and neurologic changes may be irreversible if the poisoning is severe. Toxicity develops in people who work in industry involving mercury, such as vacuum pump or thermometer manufacturing.

Aluminum poisoning develops after industrial exposure or in patients with chronic renal failure. Renal failure can cause hyperphosphatemia. One treatment for hyperphosphatemia has been aluminum-containing antacids. Absorption of aluminum (in the antacid) through the GI tract can cause aluminum poisoning. The mental status changes consist of a speech disorder followed by progressive dementia. Eventually, aluminum poisoning causes coma and death. Other systemic changes are osteodystrophy and myoclonus. The best treatment is prevention by monitoring aluminum intake (both orally and in the dialysate).

Manganese intoxication occurs occasionally in people who manufacture batteries. Mental status changes initially are limited to irritability. With chronic manganese poisoning, emotional lability, impulsiveness, and even periodic aggressiveness can develop. Manganese can cause lesions of the basal ganglia and may cause extrapyramidal signs and symptoms on physical examination. Such patients may also have masked facies and a loss of equilibrium. Unfortunately, the current treatments for manganese poisoning, levodopa and chelation with EDTA, provide limited benefit.

Arsenic poisoning, of course, can cause death in an acute overdose. However, chronic arsenic poisoning is likely to cause the gradual onset of symptoms of inflamed mucous membranes and a dermatitis. Mental status changes would mainly consist of increased lethargy and withdrawal. Severe, chronic arsenic poisoning leads to encephalopathy with marked diminution in intellectual functioning. Arsenic is found in rodenticides, insecticides, movies, and novels. The treatment is the chelating agent, B.A.L. (dimercaprol).

Bromides, found in old-time medicinal preparations, can cause syndromes that closely resemble psychiatric illness, including delirium and schizophrenia-like illnesses. Hallucinations can occur with an otherwise normal mental status exam. Neurologic symptoms can occur, too, including ataxia, sluggish pupils, and tremor. The treatment is supportive.

Why so much time and energy on conditions that are so uncommon? Two reasons. First, as you can see, these heavy metals can mimic psychiatric illness. Second, you're in a good position to one-up your attending or resident, now.

E: Endocrine Disorders

Cushing's disease can present with a variety of mental status changes. The patient may describe feeling moody with periods of euphoria alternating with periods of depression. Occasionally, a patient with Cushing's disease will present with a delirium. Patients on exogenous steroids are at risk for developing these symptoms, too.

The physical changes in Cushing's disease should be familiar to you. There is a movement of fat centrally so that a buffalo hump and obesity develop. Bones may become brittle, and the patient may become hypertensive. Diabetes can develop. The mental status changes can precede the physical stigmata of Cushing's disease.

Addison's disease can present as withdrawal, apathy, and depression. Addison's disease can cause weight loss and vomiting, so it can parade as anorexia nervosa. However, Addison's disease occurs at all ages, has the same incidence in men as women, and does not cause orange skin discoloration. Patients with Addison's disease are weak, have electrolyte abnormalities, and may have increased pigmentation if the condition is chronic.

Hyperthyroidism also can cause mental status changes, or changes in the patient's behavior. Patients so afflicted can develop hyperactivity, pressured speech, and a type of "mania." They may also suffer from increased irritability and impulsiveness. Obviously, most patients with hyperthyroidism are thin, have elevated vital signs, and have the biochemical changes associated with hyperthyroidism; i.e., abnormal thyroid function tests, e.g., increased T_4 or decreased TSH. Do you know which US president developed tachycardia and atrial fibrillation and was diagnosed with hyperthyroidism during his term in office?

Hypothyroidism will cause depression in some patients. In addition, chronic hypothyroidism can cause withdrawal, apathy, and lack of interest in previously enjoyed activities. Such patients have wasting of the lateral margins of their eyebrows, obesity, diminished basal metabolic rate that sometimes causes depressed vital signs, occasionally signs of myxedema, and "thick tongues." The deep tendon reflexes will be slowed (especially the return phase), helping establish this diagnosis. By the way, please do not start somebody who is depressed on thyroxine. This treatment is ineffective for depression except for the short term and can cause problems for the patient. Too much thyroxine may rev up his system and throw him into heart failure. If he has panhypopituitarism, it can cause him to have an Addisonian crisis. Thyroxine is not a psychotropic medication! (T3, however, is occasionally used to augment the partial response to an antidepressant.)

Hypoglycemia causes anxiety that may, when severe, progress to serious neurologic symptoms, including ataxia and coma.

D: Drugs

Certain prescription drugs are notorious for causing psychiatric syndromes in patients. Certain antihypertensives, especially some older ones, will often cause patients to feel depressed. *Reserpine* was likely to do this, as was *alpha-methyldopa* (Aldomet). Certain beta adrenergic blockers, especially *propranolol* (Inderal), but also *atenolol,* and others, have been associated with reports of depression in patients. Generally, if a patient reports to you a history of major depression, or if a patient is a "type A" businessperson, a beta blocker may not be the first choice of medication to treat his or her hypertension.

Histamine H2 antagonists (*cimetidine, ranitidine,* and others), now widely prescribed for the treatment of gastroesophageal reflux disease and peptic ulcer disease, can cause psychiatric symptoms, including, rarely, a toxic psychosis.

As an aside, what's another possible cause of an altered mental status in your patient with a bleeding ulcer in the intensive care unit? Answer: Acute severe blood loss could cause poor perfusion to the brain, resulting in delirium.

Any drug with anticholinergic properties can cause delirium (e.g., tricyclic antidepressants, over-the-counter sleeping pills, anti-Parkinsonian drugs, antipsychotics). Why does the octagenerian getting an eye examination become confused and combative? Answer: Somebody used eye drops with anticholinergic properties to dilate his pupils. Why does he become confused and combative when his eyes are patched following cataract surgery? Answer: Some patients, particularly the elderly, have marginally compensated mental functioning. When they lose a major source of incoming stimulation (e.g., vision), they can suffer a "mental decompensation." Other eye medications also cause psychiatric symptoms. Their use may be overlooked in the history. Beta blockers (*timolol, betaxolol*), used to treat glaucoma, undergo systemic absorption and may cause depression. *Acetazolamide* causes anorexia, lethargy, or depression in as many as 40% of users. Steroids can affect mental functioning in several ways. Some patients develop delirium. Others develop affective disorders (depression or mania). These mental status changes are usually seen with high doses of steroids (e.g., 40mg/day or more of prednisone). Any drug that significantly reduces serum sodium concentrations may cause weakness, delirium, or even psychosis; SSRIs are some of the culprits, especially in the elderly.

C: Cancer

Malignancies can cause subtle and not-so-subtle mental status changes. Pancreatic carcinomas frequently cause severe depression, which can be the presenting complaint. Certain tumors are known to have remote effects on the central nervous system. Lung carcinomas can cause a progressive dementia as well as other neurologic signs and symptoms. Pheochromocytomas can cause patients to suffer from anxiety attacks and "manic" episodes.

L: Lots of Others

We've saved a potpourri of disorders for last, but not because they're the least important. These are the ones that haunt psychiatrists the most. We'll run through these in list fashion, too. Sorry, there is no easy way of memorizing these, either.

Wilson's disease is a disorder of copper metabolism. It causes pathology in the eyes (*Kayser-Fleischer rings*), kidneys, brain, and liver. In the brain, it affects the basal ganglia, causing flapping or wing-beat tremors. Most importantly for this discussion, Wilson's disease can cause psychiatric complaints. Some patients appear to have nothing short of a classical psychoneurosis. Actually a number of such patients have been psychoanalyzed prior to the discovery of their disordered copper metabolism. Other patients develop a frank psychosis, making it easier to suspect Wilson's disease. The mental status changes usually develop in mid- to late adolescence. The treatment is chelation and is usually effective.

Acute intermittent porphyria is a disorder of porphyrin metabolism. AIP usually manifests with abdominal pain, transient neurologic symptoms, and mental status changes. The mental status changes in this disease, too, are protean. Some patients feel vaguely anxious or depressed, while others appear floridly psychotic. Anyone who has recently ingested a barbiturate who develops these symptoms has AIP until proven otherwise. But AIP can present in other situations, such as times of menses, stress, and other drug ingestions.

Huntington's chorea is a hereditary disease of the brain that usually presents with choreiform movements. An autosomal dominant, it typically presents in the third or fourth decade. Of interest here is the fact that Huntington's chorea can present as a schizophrenia-like psychosis. Sometimes this occasional presentation precedes the onset of the neurologic symptoms and complaints. Ultimately, these patients suffer from a severe and debilitating dementia. What's the diagnosis in a 32-year-old man with "schizophrenia" and tardive dyskinesia (involuntary movement disorder, often secondary to antipsychotic medications)? Answer: Probably schizophrenia with tardive dyskinesia, but be sure to take a careful family history for Huntington's chorea.

Vitamin B12 deficiency can present with a myriad of behavioral changes, including visual hallucinations, personality changes, or a dementia. The history might be positive for a Bilroth gastrointestinal procedure and no supplemental vitamins, or chronic, severe malnutrition. Neurologic signs may include weakness, numbness, and tingling of the extremities, loss of proprioception (ability to sense the direction of joint movement), and overactive reflexes.

Pellagra is caused by nicotinic acid deficiency and can be associated with insomnia and delusions. In addition to these mental status changes, the patient would most likely also have a rash, abdominal complaints, and cerebellar ataxia. The four D's of pellagra are diarrhea, dermatitis, dementia, and ... death if untreated.

Partial complex seizure disorder (*temporal lobe epilepsy*) is one of the greatest paraders. Although patients with temporal lobe seizures usually have simple automatisms or repetitive behaviors, they may also have schizophrenia-like or manic-like psychoses. When the diagnosis is suspected, do an EEG in a sleep-deprived state, using nasopharyngeal leads. If the diagnosis is still suspected, but the EEG is normal, a trial of an anticonvulsant may be indicated. If your manic-depressive patient gets better on carbamazepine, for example, he still could have a psychiatric illness. Some manic-depressives improve on this drug, which suggests that there may be some overlap between mania and temporal lobe epilepsy.

Hypercalcemia can cause almost any imaginable psychiatric symptom, as can *hypocalcemia.*

Hyponatremia can cause weakness, lethargy, and ultimately an organic psychosis (delirium with serious loss of reality testing, as noted above).

Hypokalemia causes weakness, anxiety, and depression.

Please don't be overwhelmed. Almost all of these disorders will be discovered if you perform a history and physical examination. Now it's time to go rain on the parade!

And, the president diagnosed with hyperthyroidism, after initial symptoms of tachycardia and weight loss (could have been anxiety or depression) while in office? George H.W. Bush in 1991.

CHAPTER 13. PSYCHIATRIC CONDITIONS OF CHILDHOOD

The psychological complaints and symptoms of children can be confusing. Children can be very symptomatic despite no serious psychological problems. Approximately 95% of children will develop a phobia, while 30-40% suffer night terrors. Enuresis occurs in 10% of 5-year-old boys. When do these and other problems warrant a workup and/or treatment? This chapter will help you decipher the odd array of symptoms and complaints that children present to their pediatricians, family doctors, and psychiatrists.

Here are some principles of human development to help you decide whether the cause of a child's symptom is serious:

1. Commonly, chronic exposure to stress in childhood leads to psychopathology. In contrast, exposure to an isolated traumatic event (e.g., 1 automobile accident, 1 surgical procedure) usually does not cause lasting personality changes. However, some families may react pathologically to a traumatic event for their child. They treat the child differently than before. This can cause difficulty for the child.
2. Some development in childhood occurs sequentially and inalterably. For example, it's not possible to walk before you can sit. A child's struggle for autonomy (age 2) precedes his development of more individualized interests in particular activities and goals.
3. Boys appear to be more vulnerable to developing psychopathology than girls; most childhood disorders are more common in boys with the exception of anorexia nervosa and other feeding and eating disorders.
4. Certain traumatic events in childhood can be reactivated throughout the lifespan. For example, a 3-year-old who loses a parent may become seriously depressed or anxious later in life in response to a minor loss or separation (such as attending summer camp).
5. Certain psychological symptoms are normal if they occur at the appropriate developmental phase. For example, it's normal for a 2-year-old to be oppositional. Oppositional behavior in a 9-year-old is not normal.

When a child presents with a behavior problem, the history can be important, too:

1. Is the problem chronic or acute? Long-standing problems usually are serious.
2. Is there a family history for psychiatric disorders? There is strong evidence for the contribution of genetic factors to the risk of developing

certain disorders (e.g., schizophrenia, bipolar disorder, enuresis, substance abuse).

3. How is the child being raised? Is discipline too severe?

4. Does either parent have a psychiatric disturbance? Children of depressed mothers are more likely to suffer developmental delays than children of "normal" mothers.

5. Is the behavior problem very disruptive (e.g., fighting in school)? This usually indicates a more serious problem.

6. Is there a history of divorce? Divorce adversely affects preschool age children more than older children. Chronic marital discord is probably harder on a child than divorce.

Now let's move on to the most common childhood problems.

Enuresis

Enuresis refers to wetting at a point in a child's development when he or she is physiologically capable of controlling his or her bladder (age 5). However, maturation occurs at variable rates in children. That means that a 4-year-old could have occasional loss of control of his bladder and still be within the range of normal.

It may be helpful to distinguish between primary and secondary enuresis. The former refers to wetting that has occurred continually in the child's life. The latter refers to enuresis that has developed after a period of at least a year during which the child was adequately bladder trained. *Nocturnal* enuresis is bedwetting that occurs during sleep, usually during sleep stages 3 and 4. *Diurnal* enuresis is either daytime wetting or both daytime and nighttime enuresis. This dichotomy is important because diurnal enuresis is more likely due to physical problems, and there is a combined type where the child has both nocturnal and diurnal enuresis. Nocturnal enuresis is an example of a parasomnia. *Parasomnias* are described later in this chapter.

What do you do for a child who has enuresis? Of course, you **CAP'IM.** You must explore the etiology of the enuresis, always remembering that genetic, developmental, and psychological factors may play a part.

C: *Central* nervous system problems, including frontal lobe tumors and spina bifida occulta, can cause wetting.

A: *Anatomical* derangements such as small bladder or posterior urethral valves can lead to enuresis.

P: The *psychological* factors in patients with enuresis are varied and are described below.

I: *Infections* of the urinary tract may result in enuresis.

M: *Metabolic* conditions like juvenile onset diabetes mellitus, sickle cell trait, and anemia can also cause enuresis.

The workup for enuresis is a simple one and should consist only of a careful history and urinalysis unless the history or exam suggests disorders requiring further evaluation. Always avoid invasive procedures unless absolutely indicated, because these procedures cause children psychological trauma.

Enuresis is a symptom that is self-limited. Heredity is a key factor, as the problem tends to run in families. In addition, more boys are affected than girls. Current medical opinion suggests that most children who wet the bed simply develop bladder control more slowly than other children. Psychological issues may contribute, including divorce, frequent moves, or other stressors affecting the family.

Autism Spectrum Disorder

Autism Spectrum Disorder (ASD) usually commences early in infancy and consists of abnormal development of social communication and social interaction, as well as an array of restrictive, repetitive behaviors, interests and activities. If the impairment is limited to difficulty with verbal and nonverbal communication and no restrictive, repetitive behaviors are present, then the diagnosis is *Social Communication Disorder.*

In both ASD and Social Communication Disorder, language abnormalities can include *echolalia* (the child repeats verbatim what is heard), mutism, pronoun reversals (e.g., the child uses "we" instead of "I"), and language delays. Typical responses to the environment include a pathological need for sameness. Such children, for example, might become anxious if the furniture in their classroom were rearranged. Their social development is delayed or absent. They show very little interest in other people and are usually found to have delayed or aberrant social milestones in their developmental histories. For example, such children might demonstrate no social outreach, very little smiling, and no interest in the communications of their parents.

Obviously, ASD may be a devastating illness but patients exhibit a range of impairment in social interactions and behavior. It occurs evenly across all social strata and may be slightly more common in boys than in girls. Some associated conditions include congenital infections (rubella, cytomegalovirus, etc.), hepatic encephalopathy, and even massive head trauma, which could result in a clinical picture indistinguishable from ASD. Children who are congenitally blind have a greater chance of having autistic mannerisms than other children. Complex genetic patterns of inheritance may exist in this condition. *Rett's Syndrome* consists of autistic behaviors plus acquired microcephaly and stereotyped hand movements.

ASD should no longer be considered simply a psychological disorder. These children have abnormal auditory evoked responses, decreased nystagmus in response to vestibular stimulation, and an increased frequency of grand mal seizures prior to adolescence. This suggests that there are organic difficulties in this condition.

The prognosis varies according to how much language development is present in the child and the child's IQ. The higher the IQ, the better the language, the better the prognosis.

Psychosis in Children

Although rare, children may be diagnosed with schizophrenia or other primary psychotic illnesses. More often, however, children may display prodromal psychotic symptoms. These may include a marked tendency to withdraw from social interaction, a marked disregard for appearance and hygiene, and other negative symptoms.

Night Terrors and Other Parasomnias

A *parasomnia* is a sleep disorder that occurs in the deep stages of sleep (stages 3 and 4). Roughly one third of children younger than 5 will experience 1 night terror (*Pavor Nocturnus*). A night terror is an awakening in the deep stages of sleep accompanied by loud screaming and frenetic behavior. The child's scream may be so bloodcurdling as to strike panic in the rest of the family, but the condition is normally very benign and self-limited. Occasionally, night terrors are precipitated by daytime stress. For that reason, a cursory history should be taken about these children to make sure that they are not being abused, experiencing inordinate stress, or having other difficulties. Night terrors can be distinguished from nightmares fairly easily. Nightmares have a dream associated with them, occur later in the sleep cycle because they occur with REM sleep, and usually occur in a child who can be wakened without great difficulty.

Sleep talking (somniloquy) occurs during all stages of sleep. It's nothing to worry about, but also can be precipitated by daytime stress.

As mentioned earlier, contrary to what we see in popular cartoons in which a character gracefully and aimlessly walks a tightrope while sleepwalking, this disorder in children (*somnambulism*) occasionally is dangerous. Children are not graced with acrobatic skill; they can trip and fall and hurt themselves. Children who sleepwalk should have their room secured, so that there is nothing dangerous to walk into. Otherwise, this condition is fairly benign. It, too, can be triggered by daytime stress.

Childhood Disruptive Behavior

Children with *Oppositional Defiant Disorder (ODD)* demonstrate negative, defiant, disobedient, and often hostile behavior towards adults and authority figures. These children can be extremely stubborn and continually test limits by ignoring directions, arguing, and failing to accept responsibility for personal wrongdoings. ODD kids have very low frustration tolerance and display hostility towards others by being verbally aggressive or deliberately annoying. When behaviors escalate frequently to physical aggression, these children are usually diagnosed with *Conduct Disorder (CD)*. Conduct disordered children are bullies with other children and can be physically aggressive to people and animals. They violate rules and can engage in deceit, theft, and destruction of property. Children with Conduct Disorder often develop adult *Antisocial Personality Disorder*. This section will not deal with nomenclatures for childhood aggressive behavior, but will help you to recognize childhood misconduct and to make a referral when appropriate.

Although it's difficult to call a 7-year-old a sociopath, the matrix for adult antisocial behavior is in childhood. No one develops aggressive or antisocial behavior in a vacuum. Exposure to repeated violence at home teaches children that this is an acceptable mode of behavior. When a child who has broken the law or hurt someone is brought to your attention, you should look for the following details in the family history. Look for the **VACUUM.**

V: *Violence* is often present in the family of a child who has committed an antisocial act (e.g., hurt someone, shoplifted, etc.).

A: *Alcoholism* is more common in families with children who exhibit antisocial behavior.

C: *Child abuse* is frequently found in the family.

U: *Unempathic parenting* can be hard to delineate, but often leads to antisocial behavior.

U: *Underpriviledged class* of itself does not cause antisocial behavior. However, children can learn violent behavior from their environment as well as from their family.

M: *Maternal deprivation* also may predispose to antisocial behavior. Generally, inadequately cared for children grow up feeling angry about this. Their anger can be vented in a variety of areas, including antisocial acts.

If the child has committed a serious crime, the behavior should *always* be taken seriously. If the child consistently breaks minor rules and regulations, this behavior should also be taken seriously. If the child has only 1 minor infraction and does not live in a **VACUUM**, you should send the child home without psychiatric treatment. If the child lives in a **VACUUM** and is breaking the law, 'the child is in trouble.

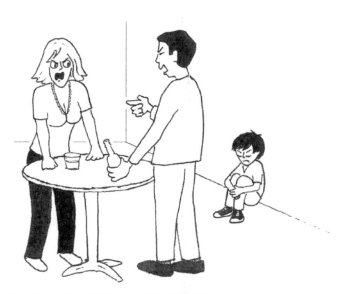

Fig. 13-1.   The child lives in a "VACUUM."

Childhood Depression and Anxiety

Children are not immune from mood and anxiety disorders. We would like to believe that children grow up happy, but this is not always the case. They can exhibit the same kinds of depressive features as their adult counterparts, with a few noteworthy exceptions.

Children are more likely to develop "*depressive equivalents*." They may be hyperactive or slightly antisocial; they may abuse drugs or fight with their family as a way of expressing an inner feeling of sadness. Usually, the child can report the subjective feeling of sadness or depression.

Disruptive Mood Dysregulation Disorder (DMDD) is a condition in which a child is chronically irritable and experiences frequent, severe temper outbursts that seem grossly out of proportion to the situation at hand. DMDD is a new disorder in DSM-5 and was created to more accurately categorize children who had previously been diagnosed with bipolar disorder. These children do not experience episodic mania or hypomania characteristic of bipolar disorder, and they do not typically develop adult bipolar disorder, although they are at elevated risk for depression and anxiety as adults.

Separation Anxiety Disorder is the most common anxiety disorder in preadolescent children. These kids feel incredible distress when separated from home, persistently worrying about harm coming to their caregivers. They may refuse to go to school and have excessive fears of being alone. Reports of nightmares involving separation are common, as are frequent somatic complaints. Children can also suffer from Pos*t-traumatic Stress Disorder* (PTSD), *Generalized Anxiety Disorder* (GAD), phobias, *Panic Disorder*, and *Obsessive Compulsive Disorder* (OCD). *Selective mutism* is an anxiety disorder that is characterized by children not speaking outside the home or only to select individuals or in select settings. While these kids understand spoken language and have the ability to speak, they have a phobia of speaking and fear of people.

Attention-Deficit/Hyperactivity Disorder

The prevalence of *Attention-Deficit/Hyperactivity Disorder (ADHD)* is about 5% in childhood and less frequent in adults. While ADHD has a neurobiological basis, environmental factors such as low birth weight or perinatal infections may play a part; the precise cause is unknown. In DSM-5 there are 3 specifiers of ADHD: predominantly inattentive presentation (easily distracted, forgetful, difficulty organizing); predominantly hyperactive/impulsive presentation (fidgety, talks out of turn, has difficulty staying in seat); or combined type. ADHD children have difficulty with executive function, and usually these problems are manifest in school and at home. They tend to suffer from low self-esteem and may have impaired social adaptive functioning.

The majority of children with ADHD will continue to have ADHD symptoms into adulthood. Adults with ADHD usually report trouble with organization, planning, task initiation, and talk completion. Overall, symptoms of inattention are much more prominent than frank hyperactivity, although adults with ADHD often report a greater sense of internal restlessness.

Intellectual Disability

Approximately 1% of the population has an *Intellectual Disability* (formerly known as *Mental Retardation*). In 35% of cases, a genetic cause can be found, and 10% are in the context of a congenital malformation syndrome (Downs Syndrome, Edwards Syndrome, Fragile X, Lesch-Nyhan, Prader Willi, Angelmans, Cri Du Chat, Fetal Alcohol Syndrome). In order to be diagnosed with an Intellectual Disability, the individual must have a very low IQ (usually below 70) in addition to impaired adaptive functioning (problems in communicating, self care, interpersonal skills, etc.).

Specific Learning Disorders

It is estimated that the prevalence of learning disabilities among children is 9.7%, making them the most common developmental disability diagnosed in childhood. Although different learning deficits commonly occur together, in the areas of reading, writing, and math, learning disabilities are coded separately. These conditions are thought to be familial and genetically based, and the risk of co-occurring anxiety, depression, and ADHD is increased. Learning disorders themselves may also secondarily cause emotional, social, and behavioral disturbance in addition to low self-esteem. Learning disorders can persist into adulthood and interfere with work and social situations. Early intervention is critical. Learning disorders do not mean that children are intellectually impaired or unable to learn; they just learn differently and usually require accommodations in order to succeed and to maximize their potential.

Tic Disorders

That's *tic*, not *tick*. A *tic* is a repetitive, purposeless movement. Eye blinking and facial grimacing are examples. Again, boys are more vulnerable. Tics are usually transient (last less than 1 year), exacerbated by stress, and more distressful to parents than patient. Tics are best treated in 2 ways. Attempt to alleviate stress and ignore the tic. If tics become chronic, psychotherapy may be indicated. Remember that tics can occur in neurologic disease, too. *Tourette's syndrome* consists of tics, impulsive behavior, and *coprolalia* (swearing). Treatment usually includes neuroleptics (major tranquilizers).

Child Abuse

We've saved the worst for last. Enormous numbers of children are abused physically and sexually every year; the effects of such abuse on the child's personality development are devastating. Physical abuse occurs in all social classes and comes in a myriad of packages, including blows, torture, and even murder. Generally, child abuse consists of any behavior within the child's environment that interferes with the child's development.

Child abuse results in personality changes in the child. These children experience a role reversal with their parents. They wind up caring for their own parents. Such abused children sometimes have precocious development. They are expected to behave like adults. For example, they may cook family meals at the age of 6. They themselves may be very aggressive at times, and when grown up will often abuse their own children. They may also suffer from developmental delays if the abuse has been severe. Such abused children may be unable to empathize with other people. Therefore, they may have difficulty appreciating the effects of violence on others.

Abused children usually are found in families where the parents, themselves, had been abused. These families are often physically isolated. The parents are suspicious of medical care and feel self-righteous in their attitudes about child-rearing. They can be very violent and may need treatment in a hospital setting. In spite of abusing their children, they may have extraordinarily high expectations of the children. Occasionally, child abuse is a disorder of neglect; it is usually a disorder of overstimulation of the child.

Recent research has emphasized collusion in child abuse. For example, one parent may dole out the physical abuse while the other "turns his or her back." The colluding parent is aware, consciously or unconsciously, that abuse is occurring, but does nothing to stop it, and may even promote it. The colluding parent is as dangerous to the child as the abusive one.

When you seriously suspect child abuse, you must report it! Report it to the social services agency and then do whatever is necessary to protect the well-being of the child. This can include hospitalization or sending the police to the home to check on the child's safety. Psychiatric treatment should usually consist of psychotherapy for both child and the family. Parental counseling is often necessary but rarely helpful in and of itself.

TREATMENT CONSIDERATIONS

Treatment of Enuresis

Enuresis is usually treated with bladder training exercises recommended by the pediatrician. Medications, usually antidepressants, may be prescribed if the child does not respond to bladder training, and a referral to a child and adolescent psychiatrist may be necessary. In any case, the treatment should also be aimed at the underlying psychological or medical condition.

Treatment of Autism Spectrum Disorders

Treatment of autism spectrum disorders should consist of a structured educational program that includes behavioral modification, encouraging social and language behaviors. Medications may be useful in cases where severe anxiety, impulsivity, or aggressive behavior is present. Psychotherapy for the family can be useful when the family is having a difficult time dealing with the child or when social and environmental factors are thought to be important in the development of the disorder in a particular child.

Treatment of Attention-Deficit/Hyperactivity Disorder

In patients with ADHD, hyperactivity and inattention severe enough to interfere with the child's functioning, either at school or at home, may require a trial of medications. Stimulant medications have been used for many years for the syndrome we now call ADHD. These include *methylphenidate* (Ritalin, and trade names), *dextroamphetamine* (Dexedrine, and others), *amphetamine/dextroamphetamine* (Adderall, and others), and other related medications. The norepinephrine reuptake inhibitor *atomoxetine* (Strattera) has also been approved by the FDA for the treatment of ADHD. Remember that all medications have side effects; use them carefully.

CHAPTER 14. THE PATIENT WITH SEXUAL PROBLEMS

An open-minded approach to the patient with sexual problems is essential. Such problems are common, arouse great anxiety and concern, and are difficult to discuss. The afflicted patient may not express his or her concerns directly. A veiled question or last-minute comment may be the only clue that the patient has something else to discuss, i.e., a sexual problem. Though discussing sexual dysfunctions may arouse anxiety in the patient as well as the doctor, they should not be overlooked. They have an important differential diagnosis and often cause significant problems in relationships. This chapter reflects the diagnostic concepts in these disorders in DSM-5 and will discuss the following types of sexual problems: *sexual dysfunctions*, *gender dysphoria*, and *paraphilic disorders*.

Sexual Dysfunctions

Frame your approach with an understanding of normal sexual physiology. Sexual *arousal* (penile erection; vaginal lubrication) may be followed by a *plateau* phase. Then, *orgasm* (ejaculation; rhythmic contractions of the perineal and perivaginal muscles) occurs. There is a refractory period after orgasm during which men are resistant to sexual excitement and cannot ejaculate, and while women may have multiple orgasms, some also may experience a refractory period. The refractory period may last a few minutes to several hours and increases with increasing age. After orgasm, *detumescence* (loss of erection/vasocongestion) occurs. Erection and vaginal lubrication are parasympathetically mediated. Ejaculation/ orgasm is mediated by the sympathetic nervous system. Therefore, awareness of injuries, drugs, or illnesses that interfere with these parts of the nervous system and determining the phase(s) in which dysfunction occurs can aid in identifying the particular sexual dysfunction.

Aside from substance or medication-induced sexual dysfunction, the sexual dysfunctions are gender specific. The 3 female dysfunctions are *female sexual interest/arousal disorder, female orgasmic disorder,* and *genito-pelvic pain/penetration disorder.* In males, the 4 diagnoses are *male hypoactive sexual desire disorder, delayed ejaculation, erectile disorder*, and *premature (early) ejaculation.*

In order to meet the criteria for a diagnosis of 1 of the sexual dysfunctions, an individual must be symptomatic for a period of 6 months (except for substance/medication-induced sexual dysfunction). The disorder must cause significant distress, may be mild, moderate, or severe, and may be further described as "lifelong versus acquired" and "generalized versus situational." Additional "associated features" may be specified, according to DSM-5, including factors related to one's partner, relationship, individual vulnerabilities, cultural or religious beliefs and medical illness.

Let's briefly review the sexual dysfunctions:

1. *Substance/medication-induced sexual dysfunction*: some common causes are alcohol, amphetamines, cocaine, sedative-hypnotic medication, and antidepressants (especially SSRIs and SNRIs).
2. *Female sexual interest/arousal disorder*: absent or reduced interest/arousal related to sexual activities, thoughts, encounters, cues, etc.
3. *Female orgasmic disorder*: delay, infrequency, or absence of orgasm or reduced intensity of orgasm sensations.
4. *Genito-pelvic pain/penetration disorder*: difficulties with a vaginal penetration during intercourse, pain during intercourse, fear or anxiety about pain or penetration, or contraction of pelvic floor muscles during sex.
5. *Male hypoactive sexual desire disorder*: persistent deficient or absent sexual thoughts, fantasies, or desires.
6. *Erectile disorder (ED)*: the failure to obtain or maintain erection during sexual activities with a partner.
7. *Delayed ejaculation*: marked difficulty or inability to achieve desired ejaculation during partnered sexual activities.
8. *Premature (early) ejaculation*: a persistent or recurrent pattern of ejaculation during partnered sexual activity within 1 minute following penetration or before individual wishes it.

TREATMENT CONSIDERATIONS

Clinical treatments have been developed for many common sexual dysfunctions. The focus is to restore sexual functioning and pleasure. All patients should initially receive a full general medical workup to rule out any underlying medical conditions or medications that may be contributing to the sexual dysfunction. Remember, the same patient may be affected by both psychological and physical factors.

Treatment of Lack of Desire

Treatment for lack of desire is a multi-step process. Clinicians can help patients identify negative attitudes and beliefs about sex, explore the origins of those ideas, and find new ways of thinking about sex. The focus then shifts to behavior changes, and the clinician also works to address any relationship problems that might exist.

Treatment of Erectile Disorder

One of the primary psychological causes of *erectile disorder (ED)* is *performance anxiety*. Therapy focuses on decreasing anxiety by taking the focus off intercourse. Sex therapists often use "sensate focus" exercises to treat ED in addition to other sexual dysfunctions. The exercises start with nonsexual touching and encourage both partners to express how they like to be touched. The goal is to help both partners understand how to recognize and communicate their preferences. For men with physical problems, physicians may prescribe medications, e.g., *sildenafil (Viagra), vardenafil (Levitra),* or *tadalafil (Cialis);* or devices (*penile prosthesis, vacuum pump*).

Treatment of Premature (Early) Ejaculation

Several techniques may be used in sexual treatment for *premature ejaculation*. Basically, the sexual activity with the partner is stopped just prior to the point where the man senses ejaculation is imminent. Then, the man either receives no stimulation or the head of the penis is squeezed by the partner. The goal of both approaches is to decrease arousal. Before the man loses his erection, the sexual activity is resumed until the man again signals the partner to stop. With this start-stop procedure, the man and his partner both gain a greater sense of control, and the problem diminishes. Anxiety plays a role in premature ejaculation. Therefore, psychotherapy frequently helps as well. Other treatments include SSRI medications and topical anesthetic ointments, such as 1% debucaine, applied to the penis.

Treatment of Painful Intercourse/Female Orgasmic Disorder

Many sex therapists prescribe the use of vaginal dilators and utilize biofeedback in the treatment of *painful intercourse/female orgasmic disorder*. Treatment can also focus on progressive muscle relaxation and cognitive behavior therapy by examining underlying beliefs that may be contributing to the pain. Female orgasmic disorder should be similarly treated. Since women differ in their responses to genital stimulation, each patient should be encouraged to explore her responses to a range of forms of stimulation (e.g., clitoral, vaginal, etc.).

Psychological factors should be explored and treated (e.g., anxiety, performance anxiety, guilt). Obviously, effective communication between sexual partners is pivotal to successful sex. Reassurance and encouragement from the primary clinician may be helpful. Some problems may be due to a lack of knowledge about sexual functioning. In these cases, books on normal sexual function may be recommended prior to psychotherapy.

Treatment of Gender Dysphoria

Gender Dysphoria is a diagnosis new to DSM-5. The term replaces *"Gender Identity Disorder "* and communicates the emotional suffering that can result from "a marked incongruence between one's experienced gender and assigned gender."

The diagnosis places emphasis on gender incongruence rather than cross-gender identification. While the condition is diagnosed by mental health providers, most of the treatment is performed by surgeons and endocrinologists. Individuals who have undergone at least one medical procedure or treatment to support the new gender reassignment are given the post-transition specifier (gender dysphoria, posttransition).

Treatment of Paraphilic Disorders

The DSM-5 chapter on paraphilic disorders includes 8 conditions: *exhibitionistic disorder, fetishistic disorder, frotteuristic disorder, pedophilic disorder, sexual masochism disorder, sexual sadism disorder, transvestic disorder,* and *voyeuristic disorder.* To be diagnosed with one of these disorders, the individual must feel "personal distress about their interest or cause functional impairment," or "the paraphilia inherently involves individuals who are nonconsenting and who have been used to gratify the paraphilia in real life and not just in fantasy." The distinction between paraphilias and other disorders reflects the idea that many people may practice atypical sexual behaviors without meriting a diagnosis of mental illness.

Paraphilias are a group of disorders in which intercourse is not the preferred means of sexual gratification. Here, we'll discuss *exhibitionism, sadomasochism, pedophilia,* and *transvestism.* Patients with these conditions don't seek help themselves unless they feel guilty about their desires. They are usually referred by courts (pedophiles, exhibitionists). Patients often have more than 1 paraphilia, e.g., a pedophile may also be an exhibitionist.

Exhibitionists derive sexual gratification (including orgasm) from exposing their genitals. The condition is more common in men who expose themselves to women and scare them. These men achieve unconscious validation that they are "men" by the reactions they obtain. Usually, exhibitionists come to the psychiatrist's attention via court referral. They are difficult to treat because they deny having the condition and don't want to change, but with intensive cognitive-behavioral therapy and legal sanctions, progress may be made.

Sadomasochists must hurt or be hurt to obtain sexual gratification. A fusion of sexual and aggressive impulses has occurred. Treatment is prolonged psychotherapy.

Pedophiles obtain sexual gratification by molesting pre-adolescent children. The victim may be a boy or girl. Treatment is, again, intensive cognitive-behavioral therapy and legal sanctions.

Transvestites are individuals who are sexually aroused by wearing clothing of the opposite gender. Treatment is long-term psychotherapy.

CHAPTER 15.   PERSONALITY DISORDERS

Everyone has a personality "style." Only a few have personality disorders. A personality disorder is a rigid, maladaptive and lasting pattern of thinking, feeling, and behaving that causes significant dysfunction in many spheres of life. A personality disorder should be distinguished from personality traits. We all have personality traits, which are behaviors or mannerisms that are habits but are not pervasive enough to be a full-blown personality disorder.

While the onset of a personality disorder generally occurs in late adolescence or early adulthood, personality disorders are usually not diagnosed before age 18. This is because the diagnosis carries stigma within both society and the medical field. Most people with personality disorders have great difficulty in learning new ways of relating to the self and the world. These conditions are extremely difficult to treat and are known to be ego-syntonic as opposed to ego-dystonic. *Ego-syntonic conditions* (which include many of the personality disorders and eating disorders) are those in which a person's thoughts, feelings, values, and behaviors are generally in harmony with "who they are." These patients often attribute symptoms and dysfunction to others. They are not likely to be distressed by their condition and often never seek treatment. In contrast, *ego-dystonic conditions* (which include anxiety disorders and mood disorders) are those in which a person's thoughts, feelings, values and behaviors are in conflict, considered unacceptable, or distressing with respect to a person's ideal self-image. Psychotherapy is the treatment of choice for all personality disorders, and medications are usually used for comorbid (co-occuring) mood, anxiety, or psychotic symptoms.

People with personality disorders may be in frequent trouble with relationships, with the law, and/or with their work. They are in **BAD SHAPE**, a mnemonic to help you remember the categories of personality disorders.

Borderline: These patients dread separations. See below for further explanation.
Antisocial: These patients habitually violate the rights and feelings of others.
Dependent: These patients rely excessively on others for guidance and emotional support.
Schizoid: These patients are aloof, withdrawn, and difficult to engage.

Schizotypal patients have odd and nearly psychotic mannerisms but aren't fully schizophrenic.

Histrionic: These patients exaggerate and respond with strong emotions to relatively minor difficulties.

Avoidant: These patients show attachment to others but shy away from social relationships. Do not confuse these patients with Schizoid personality disorder patients (who have no desire to be with others).

Paranoid: These patients are suspicious of others but not psychotic.

Passive-Aggressive: These patients use passivity to express angry feelings. For example, they may show up late for an important appointment to express their anger at their doctor.

Empathic disorder: We've fudged here. The real name of this personality disorder is *Narcissistic Personality Disorder.* However, patients with this disorder cannot empathize; in fact, they often become angry if you are not able to understand them. They are also extremely vain.

In DSM-5 the personality disorders are grouped in 3 "clusters."

- *Cluster A personality disorders* are Schizoid, Schizotypal and Paranoid. These patients tend to be very odd and eccentric.
- *Cluster B personality disorders* are Borderline, Histrionic, Antisocial, and Narcissistic.
- *Cluster C personality disorders* consist of people who tend to be very fearful and anxious. Cluster C includes Dependent, Avoidant, and Obsessive-Compulsive Personality Disorder (OCPD). Do not confuse obsessive-compulsive disorder (OCD), an anxiety disorder, with someone who has OCPD. OCD is ego-dystonic, and OCPD is ego-syntonic. In OCPD, patients are preoccupied with order, control and perfectionism to a fault.

Borderline, antisocial, and narcissistic personality disorders will be discussed in greater detail below. These are the conditions that are most common in patients who seek treatment.

Borderline Personality Disorder

Every clinician will encounter and treat patients who suffer from *Borderline Personality Disorder (BPD).* These challenging patients can evoke a wide range of conflicting emotions in clinicians: from sadness, to anxiety and anger, to fear, hopelessness, and disgust. Borderline patients experience significant problems pervasively in multiple aspects of their lives. Specifically, they suffer from unstable interpersonal relationships, unstable affects (emotions), unstable sense of self, and poor impulse control (substance abuse, fighting, reckless driving, and risky sexual behavior). These patients tend to use *splitting* as a defense mechanism, which may be manifest by idealizing a doctor on one day to devaluing the same doctor following a disappointment or misunderstanding. A related manifestation of splitting may be seen in inpatient psychiatric settings, where borderline patients tend to see certain staff members as perfect and those who attempt to set limits as only there to punish them unfairly. Borderline patients fear being alone or being abandoned and can suffer from major mood shifts throughout the day.

Unstable relationships bring patients with BPD to the doctor. Such patients dread being alone; that is, they fear "separation." To avoid separation, they may try to coerce others to stay with them. For example, they may threaten or attempt suicide when faced with a separation. They quickly attach to and over-value others (e.g., the doctor). Borderline patients pose problems for the doctor-patient relationship. Initially these patients generally over-value the doctor. To control the doctor, they may threaten suicide (e.g., if not granted a request for a prescription). They may sometimes attempt to seduce the doctor. When denied their inappropriate wishes, they occasionally sue the doctor. The doctor must behave appropriately towards all patients. If a doctor thinks his patient has BPD, and he is having trouble managing the patient, a referral to a psychiatrist is indicated. If the patient refuses a referral, the doctor has 2 choices. He can seek psychiatric consultation and attempt to deal with the patient himself, or he can decline to treat the patient, if the patient is behaving inappropriately.

Patients with BPD are at high risk for self harm (cutting and self-mutilation), which can be an outlet for expressing anger, punishing themselves, and "feeling normal" in response to a dissociated state. They can feel very empty and can also present with quasi-psychosis or "micro-psychotic" experiences or dissociative states when very stressed. Patients can experience *depersonalization* (I am not real) and *derealization* (the world is not real). They can have unusual perceptions and experience nondelusional paranoia. Again, borderline patients are unable to tolerate the idea of being alone and can be very demanding and entitled. They can respond out of proportion to real or imagined abandonment and have difficulty controlling anger. Other psychiatric disorders may co-occur, such as major depressive disorder, PTSD, and substance use disorders.

Many patients with BPD have a history of being neglected, abused, or invalidated as children. Early environmental experiences play a role in the etiology of borderline personality disorder. A child who is constantly threatened with abandonment may grow up to fear separations. Some patients may be more genetically predisposed to this disorder, and biological factors play a role (e.g., abnormal neurotransmitters, frontal lobe problems, and structural brain differences).

Antisocial Personality Disorder

Antisocial Personality Disorder (ASPD) is characterized by a basic disregard for the rights of others, recurrent law breaking, and a history of antisocial behavior in childhood (e.g., shoplifting, truancy, fighting at school). This disorder will likely also fulfill the criteria for conduct disorder. In hospitals, patients with ASPD often present with demands for pain medication. Their children may be abused. They may break the law repeatedly and have a history of lying, dishonesty, stealing, cheating, conning, or being aggressive. Antisocial patients can appear extremely (but superficially) charming. The patient will say things like, "Yeah, I stole from the church, they deserved it. . .The priest was a rotten person, but I am a peaceful man and I am very religious. I would never try to hurt or steal from you, doctor. You are here to help me." Many clinicians believe that ASPD is grossly overdiagnosed in patients from poor and minority populations and underdiagnosed in patients from higher socioeconomic backgrounds. A classic description of this disorder may be found in *The Mask of Sanity* by Cleckley and, more recently, in *Snakes in Suits: When Psychopaths Go to Work,* by Babiak and Hare.

For ASPD patients, pathological parenting often causes poor conscience development. For example, a parent who condones rather than limits aggressive behavior teaches that child that fighting is okay. Genetic factors also play a role. Adopted children with an antisocial parent (biological) are at greater risk for this condition.

Narcissistic Personality Disorder

Narcissistic Personality Disorder as a diagnostic term was first officially used in DSM-III, published in 1980. While it is a relatively new diagnosis, patients with this condition have problems we all can relate to. They like attention and admiration, have a strong sense of self-importance, are sensitive to criticism, and are preoccupied with success and power. However, they also exploit others, have abnormal relationships, and lack empathy. This last symptom is the most important. Patients with this disorder are often unable to appreciate the feelings of others. Generally, a lack of empathy in the patient's upbringing causes this condition. Growing up in an understanding environment is important for healthy psychological functioning. Unempathic parents cause children to feel lonely, inferior, and misunderstood. To compensate, these children will then try harder to please others. When they grow up, they become very sensitive to criticism and misunderstanding. They compensate for their sense of inferiority by striving for greatness, but at the same time their self-esteem is fragile. Therefore, they will come to the doctor's office when they have failed to succeed or have been criticized. They will complain of depression, boredom, or empty feelings. They may describe a wish to retaliate against the person who has criticized them. A sense of failure can even lead to suicide attempts.

TREATMENT CONSIDERATIONS

Treatment of Borderline Personality Disorder

One of the most effective treatments for borderline personality pathology is *Dialectical Behavioral Therapy (DBT)* pioneered by psychologist Marsha Linehan. This intensive, evidence-based treatment consists of DBT skills group and individualized therapy. See section on psychotherapy in Chapter 16 for more information. DBT is also effective with patients with a history of self-injurious behavior, substance use disorders, or mood disorders.

Other promising psychotherapy treatments for BPD patients include *Transference Focused Psychotherapy*, *Cognitive Behavior Therapy (CBT* or *Schema Therapy)*, and *Mentalization-Based Therapy*. The initial research evidence for these treatment approaches is encouraging. However, treatment is lengthy and complex. Feelings of abandonment may lead patients to act out in a range of ways, from unconscious and subtle to overtly conscious and provocative. These behaviors challenge us to develop ways of expressing empathy while being mindful of consistently setting boundaries and limits. The therapist must anticipate difficult times for the patient (e.g., the therapist goes on vacation, a separation) and help the patient find new ways of coping with these experiences. Some of the more severe cases will likely require hospitalization for suicidal ideation or attempt, since these patients are at high risk for suicide.

Psychotropic medications are only modestly effective. The best evidence is for using serotonin selective reuptake inhibitors (SSRIs), although mood stabilizers may be useful to treat symptoms of impulsivity and emotional lability. The medications for drug or alcohol craving in comorbid substance abuse, including *naltrexone* and *acamprosate*, may be helpful in these patients. Perceptual or cognitive disorganization problems may benefit from low dose antipsychotic agents. Fortunately, studies have shown that as the patient ages, there tends to be substantial improvement in symptoms.

Treatment of Antisocial Personality Disorder

Treatment consists of limiting the antisocial behavior, when possible. This can sometimes be accomplished with a jail term or other social pressure (e.g., taking away custody of children, if they are abused). Patients with ASPD have low self-esteem. They also react angrily when confronted. The therapist should appear to be particularly interested in these patients (helps self-esteem) and should gently confront lying, stealing, etc.

The approach to psychotherapy with these patients is similar to those with borderline personality (see above).

Treatment of Narcissistic Personality Disorder

The treatment for narcissistic personality disorder is long-term psychotherapy, similar to the treatment approaches to borderline personality. The therapist will invariably, but not deliberately, misunderstand the patient from time to time. The patient's reactions to this misunderstanding are explored and explained to him or her. Eventually, such patients come to terms with their vulnerability to criticism.

Remember, patients with a severe personality disorder are in **BAD SHAPE.** This means, they are frequently in trouble, and the trouble will significantly interfere with their life, their social relationships, their work, and even their ability to be a law-abiding citizen.

CHAPTER 16. TREATMENT MODALITIES

Psychotherapy

An exhaustive list of all psychotherapeutic treatments is outside the scope of this book, so we will focus on some of the more widely practiced approaches and orientations. While psychotherapy has likely been informally practiced since the beginning of time, Sigmund Freud, a neurologist in Vienna at the turn of the 20th century, was one of the early pioneers in psychotherapy and began to develop psychoanalysis. In today's society, most practitioners (including psychiatrists, psychologists, clinical social workers, and marriage and family therapists) use several approaches in their work and alter their approach based on the needs of the patient.

Research in psychotherapy has shown that therapeutic success in therapy across a variety of treatment approaches and clinical issues is associated with a strong *therapeutic alliance*. The therapeutic alliance may be defined as the development of a bond between the clinician and patient that feels safe and trusting, and the two participants establish mutually agreed upon tasks and goals. The therapeutic alliance has also been described as "the ability to work purposefully together."

There is strong evidence that psychotherapy can be effective and can lead people to live healthier and more productive lives. Susan Lazar in her book, *Psychotherapy Is Worth It: A Comprehensive Review of Its Cost-effectiveness,* argues that receiving more therapy for a longer period of time decreases the likelihood of having a substance use disorder, going to jail, taking time off from work, and being physically ill.

Freud's Topological Model and His Structural Model

In the late 19th century Freud became interested in neurological conditions for which there were no apparent neurologic or neuropathologic underpinnings. The diagnostic term for these patients at that time was *hysteria,* and their unexplained weakness or paralysis was called a *hysterical conversion* symptom. He decided to attempt hypnosis on them, and he discovered that these patients frequently repressed (forgot) their memories of traumatic childhood events. Freud also learned that, as adults, these patients re-enacted these repressed memories in conflict-symptom constellations; that is, they lived out and repeated these memories in maladaptive ways in an effort to master the childhood experience. Freud's *topological model* focuses on the division between the unconscious and conscious parts of the mind. The content of our unconscious minds is inaccessible to us; this is where our forbidden wishes and impulses stay safely outside of our awareness. We are capable of accessing thoughts, memories, and wishes when they are in the pre-conscious mind. There is no block between the pre-conscious and conscious, and when we do become aware of our thoughts, memories, and wishes, they become part of the conscious mind.

The development of Freud's *structural model* reflected his growing interest in how mental content was divided. To his topological model, Freud added the concepts of the *id*, the *ego*, and the *superego*. These three parts of the human psyche were the central tenets of his structural theory. Psychiatric usage of the term *ego* should not be confused with common usage, which connotes self-love or selfishness. The *id* seeks immediate pleasure and consists of aggressive and sexual wishes, known as drives. The id is impulsive and primal and can be conscious or unconscious. In contrast, the *superego* is highly moral and represents the conscience. It is the job of the rational *ego* to find balance between the id and the superego.

Ego-Defense Mechanisms

In psychiatry and psychology, viewed from the psychoanalytic perspective, the word *conflict* refers not to a conflict of the Arab-Israeli variety, but rather one that occurs in an individual's mind. When our ego feels overburdened with the conflicting demands of the id and superego, we use *defense mechanisms* (see examples below) to deal with the related feelings of anxiety and guilt and to help us handle uncomfortable emotions.

To help us remember some defense mechanisms, we can consider the following example:

> A third-year medical student is anxious to kick up her heels on Friday evening when her intern or resident suggests that they go see an interesting patient. This is the fourth time this week she's been held 2 hours late for "an interesting patient."

The conflict is that the medical student would like to slug the resident but is obliged to hold back. To strike the resident would be relatively uncivilized and contrary to what the average student has learned about dealing with other human beings. How does the psyche deal with the wish and the prohibition against the wish, both of which are in "conflict" with each other? This is where defense mechanisms often come into play.

- Hitting the resident would be considered *acting out,* and if after hitting the resident, she started to care for the resident and clean his wounds and be supportive, this would be considered *undoing.*
- If the medical student says that "all residents are bad" and "all medical students are good," this would be an example of *splitting.*

- On the other hand, she may glumly accompany the resident, and a few years later pull the same stunt on her medical student. This would be termed *identification with the aggressor!*
- If the medical student wants to slug the resident, raises her arm and fist, and then develops a psychogenic paralysis of the arm, this is a *conversion* symptom. A somatic symptom is now being used to defend against the wish to slug a superior. If the medical student were hypnotized, this buried aggressive wish would possibly be brought to the surface.

You must be wondering why hypnosis isn't the treatment of choice, then, for all of these intrapsychic disorders. Although Freud found that hypnosis could frequently uncover the buried conflict and memory, he found that psychoanalysis, a technique that involves a detailed interaction between patient and physician, was more effective in treating emotional conditions. He discovered that the best way to cure conversion or hysterical symptoms, which were very common in 19th century Europe, was to unravel, decode, and understand the myriad of defense mechanisms and resistances in his patients. Freud also encouraged patients to use free association (spontaneous, uncensored talking by the patient about whatever comes to their mind).

Terms such as *transference, countertransference,* and countless more have emerged from psychoanalysis. See below for definitions.

- *Transference* describes the unconscious feelings that the patient has towards the therapist, based on previous relationships (e.g., the therapist unconsciously reminds the patient of his own father).
- *Countertransference* describes feelings that are elicited in the clinician from being in the presence of a particular patient. These feelings can be good, bad, or mixed, and can influence care. The psychotherapist can utilize the phenomenon of countertransference as a therapeutic tool to help the patient understand emotional problems and their origins.

Psychoanalysis Today

Since the time of Freud, psychoanalysis has continued to develop, and many different theoretical orientations have emerged, including *interpersonal psychoanalysis* (inspired by the work of Harry Stack Sullivan) and *relational psychoanalysis* (introduced by Stephen Mitchell). Both interpersonal and relational psychoanalysis spend a significant amount of time exploring the relationship between the clinician and the patient. Some practitioners continue to identify as *classical* or *Freudian psychoanalysts*. Gaining a deep understanding of the different types of psychoanalysis and theories is outside the scope of this book. While psychoanalysis is widely caricatured and misunderstood, this type of psychotherapy can have powerful effects and can help people to see themselves and the world in more adaptive and healthy ways.

(See Appendix for suggested readings.)

Major Psychotherapies

Today, most psychotherapies may be broadly categorized as *psychodynamic* (focused on resolution of intrapsychic conflict and based on many principles of psychoanalysis) or *cognitive-behavioral* (focused on examining and challenging distorted and maladaptive thoughts and beliefs that can affect feelings and behaviors; or focusing on behavior change as a means to psychological change). Other types of psychotherapy we will briefly discuss include *humanistic therapy (client-centered/gestalt/existential)* and *group/family/couples* therapy.

Psychodynamic Psychotherapy

Psychodynamic Psychotherapy attempts to understand intra-psychic conflict and is based on many of the principles of psychoanalysis. This type of therapy can be short term or long term. In this form of therapy, the therapist uses both supportive and uncovering techniques to help the patient with his or her problems. The relationship between the clinician and patient is often explored, and ideas like transference, countertransference, and enactments are examined (see above). Psychodynamic psychotherapy is most useful for patients who have good levels of distress tolerance and are not psychotic or suffering from dementia.

The goals of psychodynamic psychotherapy are to gain a better sense of self and have better relationships with others. In addition to providing symptom relief, the goal of psychodynamic psychotherapy is to help the patient to develop improved self-esteem and learn to embrace life more fully in love, work, and play. In this type of therapy, the clinician also explores unconscious fantasy and dreams. The idea is that through interpretation, the therapeutic alliance, and the handling of transference, the patient will gain insight and awareness and get better.

Some forms of psychodynamic psychotherapy have undergone considerable research including *Mentalization-Based Therapy* (developed by Peter Fonagy and Anthony Bateman) and *Transference-Focused Psychotherapy* (developed by Otto Kernberg, John Clarkin and colleagues).

Cognitive Behavioral Therapy

Behavioral Therapy and Cognitive Therapy developed independently and to some extent in reaction to psychoanalytic therapy. The father of *Cognitive Behavioral Therapy* (CBT) is Aaron T. Beck. Beck began to develop cognitive therapy in the early 1960's. Other major contributors to the practice of CBT as we know it today include Albert Ellis and B.F Skinner. Ellis formulated his ideas along similar lines and termed the treatment *Rational Emotive Behavior Therapy (REBT)*. Skinner began to theorize on learning theory and behavioral theory much earlier.

We will first review some basic *learning theory* ideas and then move on to important principles and concepts of CBT that you should become familiar with.

In *learning theory*, psychological symptoms are considered to be the result of learned or, more specifically, conditioned maladaptive patterns of response that develop over time, based on the contingencies and rewards or consequences associated with human action. In treatment, a particular behavior or response is identified for the focus of therapeutic intervention.

Behavioral therapy (based on learning theory) tries to change problematic behavior or teach new adaptive behavior through 2 basic principles of behavioral change: classical conditioning and operant conditioning.

Classical conditioning, most associated with Ivan Pavlov, deals with training a reflex; *operant conditioning* deals with the modification of voluntary behavior. *Conditioning* means that we are trying to associate or connect something new with an old relationship.

In classical conditioning, an *unconditioned stimulus* is a thing that naturally elicits a response. When a dog sees food (seeing food = *unconditioned stimulus),* it starts to salivate (salivation = *unconditioned response*). This is an example of an unconditioned relationship; it happens naturally and automatically. If we present a new stimulus not previously associated with a response, such as the ringing of a bell (a *conditioning stimulus*), at the same time that we present the old stimulus (food = unconditioned response), we can eventually establish a new conditioned relationship, because the dog will eventually start to salivate when it hears the bell, even before it can see the food. This new conditioned stimulus-response relationship was created by associating a new stimulus with an old unconditioned stimulus-response pattern.

Systematic desensitization tries to eliminate an unwanted conditioned response like anxiety by gradually exposing the patient to the associated conditioned stimulus in a relaxing situation. *Flooding* occurs when the person is presented with intense exposure to the stimulus in an attempt to eliminate the unwanted conditioned response.

In *operant conditioning* (coined by B.F. Skinner), the patient learns that behaviors have consequences, and rewards and punishment are used to attempt to change behavior.

Psychotherapeutic interventions associated with classical conditioning include systematic desensitization and exposure therapy, which are often used to treat PTSD, phobias, panic disorder, and related anxiety disorders. Interventions associated with operant conditioning include applied behavior analysis (observation and measurement of behaviors) and token economy (rewarding patients for desirable behaviors).

Cognitive behavioral therapy (CBT) is designed to be time-sensitive, educative, and goal directed. CBT tends to focus more on the "here and now" rather than on the past and early personal experiences. CBT dedicates a lot of time to teaching patients skills to examine their own thoughts and change their unhelpful behavior. Overall, CBT posits that:

- How we think influences how we feel (physically and emotionally), which influences how we behave, the decisions we make, and the life we live.
- *Automatic thoughts* are thoughts and images that jump into the person's mind without effort or choice. Persistent patterns of themes in individuals'

thoughts reflect their basic beliefs about the self, the world, and others, as well as core ways of perceiving the past, present, and future. These deeper levels of cognition, called *core beliefs* or *schemas*, influence individuals' perceptions.

- One of the main things that the cognitive model focuses on is "distortions in thinking." Patients learn that just because they think something, it does not mean that the thought is 100% true. Patients are taught skills to evaluate their thinking and to see for themselves if and how much of a thought is true. Patients are given skills and empowered to not feel so helpless in the face of negative thoughts.
- The initial assessment of the patient focuses on eliciting the distorted or maladaptive thoughts, beliefs, and behaviors that are contributing to and maintaining the patient's depression, anxiety or other condition.
- In learning or cognitive behavioral theory, psychological symptoms are considered to be the result of learned or conditioned maladaptive patterns of response that develop over time based on the contingencies and rewards or consequences associated with human action.

In treatment, a particular behavior or response is identified for the focus of therapeutic intervention. In practice, techniques based on the cognitive model and learning theory are used together. CBT sessions are structured, and mutually agreed-upon "homework" is assigned to the patient. Elements of the CBT sessions and homework may include identifying and responding to automatic thoughts and cognitive distortions, making activity schedules, exposure, evaluating and systematically examining maladaptive beliefs, training in assertiveness and in progressive muscle relaxation, etc. "Role playing" with the therapist is also a big part of CBT and can help patients to identify automatic thoughts and resulting emotions and also to practice new behaviors, such as social skills. A lot of time in CBT is spent on relapse prevention (helping the patient to identify the early warning signs of illness and what to do about it, including the use of specific CBT techniques).

An excellent text for learning more is *Cognitive Behavior Therapy: Basics and Beyond* (2011) by Judith S. Beck, PhD. While some refer to CBT as the "second wave" of behavior therapy, other behavioral therapies known as "third wave" have emerged and embrace *mindfulness* and acceptance from eastern thinking. While there is no universally agreed on definition of mindfulness, it is helpful to understand the concept as embracing humanness and accepting one's body, thoughts, feelings, and emotions without judgment. Jon Kabat-Zinn has described mindfulness as "paying attention, in a particular way, on purpose, to just the current moment, nonjudgmentally."

Other "Third-Wave" Therapies

These "third wave" therapies include Marsha Linehan's *Dialectical Behavior Therapy (DBT)*, which will be described below. In the suggested reading list in Appendix A, you will also find references to Steven Hayes, Kirk Strosahl, and Kelly Wilson's *Acceptance and Commitment Therapy (ACT)*, Jon Kabat-Zinn's

Mindfulness-Based Stress Reduction (MBSR), and Zindel Segal, Mark Williams and John Teasdale's *Mindfulness-Based Cognitive Therapy (MBCT)*.

Dialectical Behavior Therapy is a comprehensive treatment, developed by Marsha Linehan, PhD, which includes individual therapy, skills groups, and coaching in between these sessions. The clinician is also part of a greater consultation team with other clinicians. Some of the techniques are borrowed from CBT. In DBT, patients work to resolve the seemingly oppositional or dialectical ideas of "self-acceptance" and "change" to promote relief and growth. There is an emphasis on validation and the patient works on "accepting" distressful thoughts, feelings, and behaviors rather than struggling with them to gain coping skills over 4 modules including:

1. Mindfulness (based on Buddhist meditative practices)
2. Emotion regulation
3. Distress tolerance
4. Interpersonal effectiveness

DBT patients must adhere to a very strict contract and are not allowed to talk about very emotionally charged material or suicidal behavior in groups. Difficult and personal topics are reserved for individual therapy sessions.

Existential-Humanistic Psychotherapies represent a broad range of therapeutic approaches that embrace the concept of freedom and responsibility and try to work on the whole person, including mind, body, and spirit. Patients work to free themselves from self-imposed limitations and come to a deeper understanding of their authentic life goals versus those imposed by others or by a rigid sense of self. Concern and respect for others are also important themes that are stressed. The best-known theorist associated with existential-humanistic psychotherapy is Abraham Maslow. Maslow believed that our motivations in life are solely based on our needs. Maslow said that we have many different types of needs, and their importance to us changes throughout our lives. Several specific types of therapy derived from this perspective are briefly described here:

Person-Centered Therapy was developed by Carl Rogers, who moved away being "an authority" on the patient's inner experiences. He believed that patients are in the best position to resolve their problems if the clinician can provide a warm, accepting, and safe environment in which the individual feels free to talk about issues and can gain understanding and insight into them. This type of therapy is nondirective, and clinicians NEVER tell their clients what to do. Techniques are not of crucial importance.

Existential Psychotherapy focuses on free will, self-determination, and the search for meaning. Therapy primarily focuses on the 4 "existential problems" considered to be at the root of most psychological difficulties: fear of death, freedom vs. responsibility, isolation, and meaninglessness. The names most associated with Existential Psychotherapy (not Existential Philosophers like Sartre and Kierkegaard) are Rollo May, James Bugental, and Irvin Yalom.

Gestalt Therapy was developed largely by Fritz Perls. There is an emphasis on the idea of "organismic holism," the importance of being aware of the "here and now" and accepting responsibility for yourself. Techniques include confrontation, role-playing, and dialogue between two parts of a personality. Gestalt therapists also stress the importance of the present because one can best appreciate the totality of an experience as it occurs.

Other Therapies That May Draw on Multiple Orientations

Motivational Interviewing (MI) was developed and initially studied by William Miller and Stephen Rollnick. MI involves paying very close attention to the natural language about change that patients use. MI is a collaborative conversation between a patient and clinician that addresses ambivalence about change. The theory of MI is that people talk themselves into change, based on their own values and interests. MI is designed to help patients mobilize their strength, commitment, and personal resources for transformation. In addition, MI embodies acceptance and compassion, and has been described as a "way of being." The 5 communication skills that clinicians use are open questioning, affirming, reflecting, summarizing, and informing. MI can be used as a stand-alone treatment or sprinkled onto CBT and psychodynamic therapies in addition to a wide variety of other therapeutic orientations. It is often used in patients with substance use disorders.

Interpersonal Psychotherapy (IPT) is a short-term treatment shown to be effective for treating primarily depression. It was developed by Gerald Klerman, and Myrna Weissman. IPT focuses on the "here and now" and sets out to improve interpersonal relationships that contribute to depression. The 4 basic problem areas recognized by IPT are:

- *Unresolved grief.* In normal bereavement, the person usually begins to return to normal functioning within a few months. Unresolved grief is generally grief that is either delayed and experienced long after the loss, or distorted grief, in which the person may not feel emotions but instead experiences other symptoms.
- *Role disputes.* Role disputes occur when the patient and significant people in his or her life have different expectations about their relationship.
- *Role transitions.* Depression may occur during life transitions (retirement, career change, etc.) when a person's role changes and he or she doesn't know how to cope with the change.
- *Interpersonal deficits.* This may be an area of focus if the patient has a history of inadequate or unsupportive interpersonal relationships.

Group Therapy. Group therapists draw on many theoretical backgrounds. Psychotherapy groups are commonly used in clinic settings and may be used to help patients develop social skills. They are particularly useful for patients with chronic maladaptive personality traits and interpersonal conflicts. Groups are also common for patients with chronic mental illnesses, with substance use disorders, and occasionally in other situations. Groups may provide interpersonal support, which can enhance self-esteem among the members via an awareness that other people suffer from the same symptoms, feelings, and thoughts. When treating children, family or couples therapy can be extremely important in helping alter feelings and behavior that may adversely affect the child.

Family Therapy. As with group therapy, family therapy contains elements from various schools of therapy. Simply including the family in the assessment, decision-making and treatment planning for the patient results in better patient adherence and improved outcome. Including families does not require any specific training and can occur as a routine part of care.

There are a variety of evidence-based family interventions that provide education to families, allow family members the opportunity to express their feelings and discuss their difficulties managing the illness. Multifamily psychoeducational group treatment is especially helpful, since families learn from each other. Psychoeducation explores the meaning of the illness for each family member and helps the family develop a good repertoire of coping skills.

Family Systems Therapy focuses on interrupting negative interpersonal behavior patterns and promoting alternative, positive patterns. Family systems therapy generally requires considerably more training than family psychoeducation and is usually provided by family therapists who are not physicians. Other evidence-based family therapies use cognitive behavior therapy and psychodynamic concepts and techniques to help family members change in productive ways.

PSYCHOPHARMACOLOGY

Antidepressants

Antidepressants are probably the most widely prescribed psychotropic agents, so we'll discuss them first. Many antidepressants have significant antianxiety, as well as antidepressant, effects. In fact, they have FDA "indications" for more anxiety disorders than they do for depressive disorders.

There are 4 main classes of antidepressant drugs:

1. *tricyclic antidepressants (TCAs)*
2. *monoamine oxidase inhibitors (MAOIs)*
3. *selective serotonin reuptake inhibitors (SSRIs)*
4. *serotonin norepinephrine reuptake inhibitors (SNRIs)*

*Imipramine (*Tofranil*)*, the first tricyclic antidepressant, was developed in the late 1950's. Since that time, *amitriptyline (*Elavil*)*, *doxepin (*Sinequan*)*, *desipramine (*Norpramin*)*, and others have been developed. A proposed mechanism for the effectiveness of these drugs is based on their effect on the release, uptake, or metabolism of norepinephrine or serotonin in the central nervous system. Although many new antidepressants have been developed, there has yet to be conclusive proof that any of the newer drugs are significantly more effective than *imipramine* in treating randomly selected patients with severe depression.

SSRIs

The SSRIs became the first-line agents for both major depression and dysthymia in the 1990s due, primarily, to their low side effect profile compared to the TCAs and MAOIs. Several of them are also indicated for one or more of the following: panic disorder; obsessive compulsive disorder; social anxiety disorder; generalized anxiety disorder; and post-traumatic stress disorder. *Fluoxetine* *(Prozac)* was introduced in 1988 and is still the most well-known antidepressant in the country. The favorable side effect profile and relative safety (lower toxicity in overdose) and simplicity has led to a dramatic rise in SSRI use. Most SSRIs are minimally anticholinergic and antihistaminic. Therefore, dry mouth, constipation, blurred vision, and urinary retention are uncommon. *Paroxetine (Paxil)* appears to be the most anticholinergic and may cause some of these problems. Recently, gradual weight gain has been more frequently reported with all of these agents, though again, *paroxetine* may be the worst offender.

All of the SSRIs may cause nausea, tension headaches, increased anxiety, insomnia (though paradoxically they may cause daytime drowsiness), and sexual dysfunction. Decreased libido, anorgasmia in women, and delayed ejaculation in men may occur in 20–40% of patients. *Bupropion* or *buspirone* (psychotropic agents to be discussed later) may be helpful for this side effect. *Sildenafil* (Viagra), *vardenafil* (Levitra), or *tadalafil* (Cialis), medications approved for erectile dysfunction in men, are now often prescribed for the sexual side effects of the SSRIs and may be helpful in some patients. Controlled studies do not support their use in women, but many clinicians report that these agents do work in some women as well as some men.

Hyponatremia has been reported in older patients on SSRIs and should be considered in patients on SSRIs who have an altered mental status. An increased risk of bruising, prolonged bleeding time, and gastrointestinal (GI) bleeding are uncommon but important potential side effects of SSRIs. When used in conjunction with nonsteroidal anti-inflammatory drugs (NSAIDs), the risk of GI bleeding is further increased.

In 2004, the FDA issued a warning concerning the use of antidepressants, including the SSRIs, in children and adolescents. The British and the European Union have issued similar, and in some cases, more restrictive warnings concerning antidepressants in young people (those under the age of 25). These decisions have been based on retrospective reviews of many original efficacy studies focusing on the occurrence of suicidal ideation allegedly caused by these agents. Most US psychiatrists continue to believe that the overwhelming evidence is that the SSRIs are extremely safe and, in fact, have led to lower suicide rates. The SSRIs are not cardiotoxic and are rarely, if ever, lethal in overdose when no other drugs are involved. Only 10–15% of patients discontinue these agents due to side effects.

There are now multiple SSRIs approved for adults in the United States; each has advantages and dis-advantages. When beginning treatment of a patient with *major depression* or *persistent depressive disorder* here are some of the issues to consider. All of the SSRIs are basically equally effective for these indications except *fluvoxamine*, which is only approved for obsessive-compulsive disorder (OCD). The choice of agent rests on other considerations including side effects, drug interaction potential, elimination half-life, and cost. Six SSRIs *(fluoxetine, sertraline, paroxetine, citalopram, fluvoxamine* and *escitalopram)* are now available generically. The newer SSRI's are *vilazodone* (Viibryd) and *vortioxetine* (Trintellix).

Fluoxetine is approved for the treatment of depression in adults and children (the only SSRI to have this indication). It also has indications for OCD, premenstrual dysphoric disorder (PMDD), and bulimia nervosa. It has a half-life of 4–7 days, so occasional missed doses aren't a problem, and there are usually few withdrawal side effects upon discontinuation (in fact, Prozac Weekly, a 90mg capsule for once weekly dosing was introduced several years ago). However, *fluoxetine* is a significant inhibitor of the cytochrome (CY) P450 2D6 enzyme in the liver and may have many clinically significant drug interactions due to its effects on CYP450 2C19 as well. The typical starting dose is 10mg in the morning for 7 days then 20mg each morning. Dosing in children is based on body weight and, generally, should only be prescribed and monitored by a child psychiatrist or pediatric neurologist. Some response may occur within a few days. Most patients who respond have some improvement in 2–3 weeks, and the first follow-up visit should be scheduled in this time period. The ultimate effect of a given dose of *fluoxetine*, as with most SSRIs, may not occur for 6–8 weeks. If symptoms are severe and there is only a partial response at the first follow-up visit, many clinicians increase the dose by 50–100%. The usual daily adult dose is 20–40mg.

Sertraline (Zoloft) has indications for depression, panic disorder, post-traumatic stress disorder (PTSD), social phobia (or social anxiety disorder), premenstrual dysphoric disorder (PMDD), and OCD in adults. It is indicated for OCD in children. *Sertraline's* half-life is approximately 24 hours. It has less effect on liver enzymes than *fluoxetine* or *paroxetine*, and clinically significant drug interactions are un- common. Withdrawal side effects may occur on abrupt discontinuation. Usually the starting dose of *sertraline* is 25mg each morning. After 7 days the dose is increased to 50mg. Follow-up and dosage increases are similar to *fluoxetine*, and the most common daily dose of *sertraline* is 100mg.

Paroxetine is approved for depression, panic disorder, OCD, social phobia, PTSD, and generalized anxiety disorder (GAD). *Paroxetine* has a half-life of about 24 hours. Patients report more rapid reductions in anxiety with *paroxetine* than with the other SSRIs, but there is usually no difference after several weeks. It has several disadvantages, including more frequent sexual side effects, weight gain, and withdrawal complaints than the other agents. Withdrawal often takes several months, slowly tapering the dose. Withdrawal symptoms include dizziness, anxiety, irritability, and insomnia. In addition, *paroxetine* affects the liver's CYP450 2D6 enyzme to a similar degree as *fluoxetine*. Typically, 10mg of *paroxetine* is prescribed each morning for 1 week; then the dose is increased to 20mg daily. The average adult dose is 20–40mg.

Citalopram (Celexa) and its S isomer *escitalopram* (Lexapro) are approved by the FDA for major depression and GAD (*escitalopram* only). As with *sertraline*, they have modest effects on the liver's enzyme systems and are unlikely to cause significant drug interactions. The sexual side effects of *citalopram* are similar to those of *fluoxetine* and *sertraline*. *Escitalopram* may, indeed, be the least problematic in this regard. *Citalopram* is started at 10–20mg daily and increased to 20–40mg after 1 week. *Escitalopram* is typically begun at 5mg for 7 days, then 10mg daily.

Overall, *sertraline*, *citalopram*, and *escitalopram*, with their reduced risks for drug interactions, are the initial choice of most clinicians.

After an unsuccessful trial of an SSRI (usually 3–8 weeks), another SSRI is usually considered if there was a significant reduction in symptoms, but side effects were unacceptable. *Escitalopram* may cause less sexual side effects; *paroxetine* may cause less GI side effects; *fluoxetine* may be less sedating; *sertraline* has the most flexible dosing, with the possibility of using 12.5mg increments up to 200mg.

If fatigue, mild sedation, or sexual side effects are problematic with an otherwise effective SSRI, *bupropion* (Wellbutrin, Wellbutrin SR, and *Wellbutrin XL*), is often added. Typically, 100mg SR or 150mg XL is added each morning, and the patient is monitored closely. This regimen is sometimes effective, but additional side effects may include anxiety, irritability, and insomnia.

SNRIs

Another first-line antidepressant choice is *venlafaxine* (Effexor and Effexor XR). It was the first serotonin norepinephrine reuptake inhibitor (SNRI). At initial doses it is essentially an SSRI, but at higher doses it produces norepinephrine reuptake inhibition as well. Side effects are similar to the SSRIs. However, it may cause more initial anxiety, insomnia, and nausea, and fewer sexual side effects and problems with weight gain. Withdrawal from *venlafaxine* is frequently problematic and comparable to that of *paroxetine*. Occasionally patients require months to taper and discontinue *venlafaxine*. Some authors and the manufacturer cite studies that show increased efficacy compared to other agents. There is no consensus on this issue, and most view *venlafaxine* as equal in efficacy to the other antidepressants at comparable doses. The starting dose is 37.5mg XR each morning for 4-6 days, then 75mg for 4-6 days, then 150mg each a.m. The usual dose is 150–225mg daily.

Other medications in this class are *duloxetine* (Cymbalta), *desvenlafaxine* (Pristiq), and *levomilnacipran* (Fetzima). SNRIs are antidepressants that also may be useful for neuropathic pain, and *duloxetine* also has an FDA indication for fibromyalgia. Dosing for *duloxetine* is 30 to 120mg daily, depending on the indication. *Desvenlafaxine* is dosed at 50mg daily. *Levomilnacipran* may be started at 20mg daily and titrated to a maximum of 120mg daily.

Other Antidepressants

Bupropion is also a first-line antidepressant choice, especially in patients who exhibit "atypical" depressive symptoms. These include hypersomnia, increased appetite and weight, mood reactivity (mood improves with positive experience), and excessive fatigue. *Bupropion* affects norepinephrine and dopamine neurons but has little serotonergic action. It can cause insomnia, irritability, anxiety, and headaches but does not cause sexual side effects or weight gain. In fact, bupropion may increase libido and make weight loss easier. *Bupropion* does not usually cause the rapid calming effect associated with the SSRIs and, at first, may initially intensify affects. This is distressing for some patients but welcomed by others, who feel "numb" or "flat" with the SSRIs. The usual starting dose is 100-150mg of the SR formulation each morning. After 4–6 days the dose is increased in 100 or 150mg increments. The minimum effective dose for major depression is 300mg daily, and the maximum dosage is 450mg (400 for the SR form). The XL form may be given once daily (the older forms required bid or tid dosing). *Bupropion SR* is also indicated as an aid in smoking cessation.

Mirtazapine (Remeron) is an effective antidepressant with serotonergic and noradrenergic effects. It is sedating and may act more rapidly than the other anti-depressants. In addition to sedation, side effects include increased appetite and weight, increased serum cholesterol, and (rarely) lowered white blood cell count. Peripheral edema also occasionally occurs. *Mirtazapine* may be started at its mini-mally effective dose, 30mg each night, but many clinicians begin at 7.5-15mg hs and titrate to the effective dose. (The sedative effects are most prominent at lower doses and, when this is a consideration, some clinicians use the drug as a sedative combined with another antidepressant at a full therapeutic dose.) If there is no reduction in symptoms after 2–3 weeks, an increase to 45–60mg is appropriate. As with other antidepressants, the maximum effect may not occur for 6–8, or even 12, weeks.

Trazodone (Desyrel) is a serotonergic non-SSRI that was introduced in the late 1970s. It offered an alternative to the TCAs and MAO-Is that appeared to cause less weight gain and minimal cardiovascular effects. However, it is so sedating that it gradually became a non-addictive alternative sedative and has been rarely used as an antidepressant in recent years. The sedative dose is 25-300mg hs. The therapeutic dose for major depression is 400-600mg hs. In addition to common side effects of dry mouth, orthostasis and morning drowsiness, one unusual but important potential side effect is priapism.

Nefazodone (Serzone), a serotonergic non-SSRI and close chemical relative of *trazodone*, was introduced in the mid-1990's. Initially *nefazodone* was considered as a first-line agent with advantages that include antianxiety and sedative proper-ties plus a lack of sexual side effects and weight gain. However, *nefazodone* has been associated with severe liver toxicity leading to liver failure. The reported risk is 1 in 250,000 patient years (this is a measure sometimes used in medical research; in this example, if 125,000 patients took nefazodone for 2 years [2 x 125,000 = 250,000], 1 of the patients would develop liver failure). This has led at least one country to ban it, and the original manufacturer to withdraw it from the market. Some patients who have done very well on nefazodone prefer to continue using it, and some choose to try it because of intolerable side effects with other agents.

Vortioxetine (Brintellix) is a serotonin modulator that has effects on multiple receptors and was approved by the FDA in 2013.

As noted above, the tricyclics and MAOIs are no longer considered first-line agents but they can be very useful in certain cases.

Amitriptyline, nortriptyline, and *doxepin* are most frequently used by clinicians today for sleep in patients with the added problem of pain. In these patients the dosing is usually low, often beginning at 10mg hs and increasing to an effective dose of 30-50mg hs. The initial dosage of a tricyclic antidepressant for major depression (*imipramine, amitriptyline, nortriptyline* and *doxepin* are most commonly used today) should be 25–50mg/hs. It should be increased by 25mg every 3–4 days until the therapeutic dosage is reached (usually 150-250mg/day). Patients usually begin to respond within 2 weeks of reaching the therapeutic dose; however, response occasionally takes up to 6 weeks. In older people, antidepressants should be used cautiously, as they (like many drugs) may be metabolized more slowly, thus increasing the risk of toxicity. The danger of falling due to orthostatic hypotension calls for lower initial dosages and a slower increase in dose in this age group. Other side effects of the tricyclics may include anticholinergic and antihistamine symptoms. Cardiac arrhythmias (most commonly prolonged PR interval, but also more serious abnormalities) are possible, and this is the primary reason that the tricyclics may be lethal in overdose. These drugs are metabolized in the liver, and jaundice has occurred rarely.

Clomipramine (Anafranil) was the first medication approved for the treatment of obsessive-compulsive disorder (OCD). It is a first-generation tricyclic with a side effect profile similar to amitriptyline. Most of the SSRIs have now received indications by the FDA for OCD and are the first choice for this condition due to their favorable side effect profiles. Effective treatment for OCD usually requires medication dosages in the higher end of the accepted range as well as CBT.

The *MAO inhibitors* are also effective antidepressants. However, in addition to affecting norepinephrine and serotonin in the central nervous system, they also affect the metabolism of tyramine. A buildup of tyramine could lead to a hypertensive crisis if excess tyramine were ingested (in cheese, beer, beans, yeast). Sympathomimetic drugs (tricyclics, *ephedrine, L-dopa*, decongestants) may potentiate the MAO inhibitors' hypertensive effects. For this reason, psychiatrists have been cautious about using these drugs. Recent research has suggested that this class of drugs is effective in treating severe depressions and patients with refractory panic disorder. Major MAO inhibitor drugs include *phenelzine* (Nardil), *isocarboxazide* (Marplan), and *tranylcypromine* (Parnate).

The treatment of panic disorder often includes 1 of several antidepressants as well as cognitive behavioral therapy. Imipramine was first used for panic in the 1960s, and it is still occasionally used for this indication. The MAO inhibitors are often very effective but their use is limited due to the potential adverse reactions cited above. The SSRIs have become a first-line medication treatment for panic disorder and, though higher doses are sometimes required, occasionally patients respond to one-half of the usual dose.

The general treatment strategy for major depression is to begin with an SSRI, *bupropion, venlafaxine,* duloxetine, or *mirtazapine*; adjust the dose as appropriate; and monitor for side effects with a follow-up visit in 2–3 weeks and every 3–4 weeks thereafter until response or remission occurs. Response is usually defined as a 50% reduction in the Hamilton Depression Scale (HAM-D) score and remission as a HAM-D of 7 or less. Other evidence-based depression scales that are useful for monitoring patients include the *Beck Depression Inventory*, 2nd edition (BDI2) and the *Quick Inventory of Depressive Symptoms (QIDS)*. If there is no response or partial response to the maximum dose of a given agent, it is reasonable to make a change to an antidepressant in a different class, e.g. from an SSRI to an SNRI. An alternative in the case of a partial response to a single agent is to add *lithium carbonate* (the main evidence for this comes from studies with TCAs) or a drug from a different class, usually *bupropion, mirtazapine*, or a TCA. If a patient has a significant response to an SSRI but complains of fatigue and/or sedation, then *bupropion*, or *modafinil* (Provigil), which is a drug indicated for narcolepsy, is often added to counter these effects. The next step in treatment-resistant cases is often a trial of a TCA, with or without one of the previously tried drugs. A trial of an MAOI may then be recommended.

A course of electroconvulsive therapy (ECT) may be necessary depending on the acuity of the situation and ultimately the patient's choice. A major multisite study funded by the National Institutes of Mental Health (NIMH), the Sequenced Treatment Alternatives to Relieve Depression (STAR*D), provided a useful algorithm for decision making.

A rare but serious side effect of treatment with antidepressants is the *serotonin syndrome,* which is more likely to occur when 2 antidepressants are used concurrently, especially an SSRI and an MAOI. However, it also can occur when a drug with some MAOI properties (such as some agents for tuberculosis) or one with serotonergic effects (such as *dextromethorphan* or *tramadol*) is added to an SSRI. There have also been reports of the serotonin syndrome when the herbal drug *St. John's Wort* is added to an SSRI. The most common symptoms of this potentially lethal condition are delirium, fever, myoclonus, hyperreflexia, tremor, and ataxia.

Evidence-based practice guidelines have been developed for the treatment of major depression, bipolar disorder, schizophrenia and other psychiatric disorders. Prominent among these include the American Psychiatric Association's guidelines and the Veterans Administration's National Center for PTSD, as well as the recommendations of the NIMH.

Drug	Usual effective dose range	Sedation	Anti-anxiety effects	Anti-cholinergic effects
Fluoxetine	20-60mg/d	+	++	0
Paroxetine	20-50mg/d	++	+++	+
Sertraline	50-150mg/d	+	+++	0
Citalopram	40-80mg/d	+	++	0
Escitalopram	10-20mg/d	+	+++	0
Venlafaxine	75-225mg/d	+	++	0
Duloxetine	60-120mg/d	+	++	0
Bupropion	300-450mg/d	-	-	+

Fig. 16-1.   First-line antidepressants. For initial treatment of depression in most patients.

Antipsychotic Agents

Psychopharmacology has made major advances in the past several decades. The development of *chlorpromazine* (Thorazine) as an antipsychotic drug in the 1950's began a major change in psychiatric treatment. Since then, the ability to ameliorate some of the symptoms of chronic schizophrenia with chlorpromazine and later drugs has enabled a drastic reduction of the population in state mental hospitals.

These drugs are also called *major tranquilizers* or *neuroleptics*. The first family of these drugs was the phenothiazines in which chlorpromazine was followed by *trifluoperazine* (Stelazine), *perphenazine* (Trilafon), *thioridazine* (Mellaril) and *fluphenazine* (Prolixin). Subsequently, other antipsychotic drugs of somewhat different chemical structures were developed, including *thiothixene* (Navane), *haloperidol* (Haldol), and others. The primary indication for these drugs is schizophrenia. Other indications may be the manic phase of bipolar disorder, paranoid states, and intoxication with sympathomimetic drugs (such as amphetamines or cocaine), when delusional symptoms resembling acute schizophrenia develop.

In the 1990's a new class of antipsychotic agents appeared. This group was first called *atypical* because their predominant mechanism of action in the brain did not appear to be the blockade of dopamine (D2) receptors as is the case with the older antipsychotics. While the new drugs act at the D2 site, they also act at multiple other sites, including serotonin receptors. The first atypical antipsychotic was *clozapine* (Clozaril). It is more effective than haloperidol, the previous antipsychotic benchmark, for the positive symptoms (hallucinations and delusions) of schizophrenia, and at least as effective as haloperidol for negative symptoms (apathy, withdrawal, flat affect). These new drugs are now also called *second-generation antipsychotics (SGAs)*.

The next drug in this class, *risperidone* (Risperdal), was released more recently and appears to be as effective as haloperidol for positive and negative symptoms. The following other SGAs have been approved by the FDA: *olanzapine* (Zyprexa), *quetiapine* (Seroquel), *ziprasidone* (Geodon), *aripiprazole* (Abilify), *asenapine* (Saphris), *iloperidone* (Fanapt), *paliperidone* (Invega), *lurasidone* (Latuda), and *brexpiprazole* (Rexulti). These agents appear to be roughly equal in efficacy and have a side effect profile that offers some advantages, but also some disadvantages, compared to haloperidol. Clozapine is more effective than all other antipsychotics, including haloperidol, but a 1% risk of agranulocytosis necessitates an extensive monitoring program by psychiatrists. It is approved only for those patients whose psychotic illness has been resistant to conventional treatments.

The SGAs, particularly *olanzapine, risperidone, quetiapine* and *aripiprazole*, soon became the drugs of choice for most psychotic disorders in the early 2000's. *Paliperidone, iloperidone, asenapine*, and *lurasidone* were approved by the FDA later in the decade. The SGAs appeared to cause fewer extrapyramidal side effects than the older drugs and appeared to pose less risk for tardive dyskinesia. *Risperidone, aripiprazole*, and *lurasidone* are more physically activating for some patients. *Olanzapine* and *quetiapine* are more sedating, but all of these agents are associated with significant weight gain. *Quetiapine* was associated with the development of cataracts in some laboratory animals, and FDA recommendations are for slit lamp exams before and during the treatment. However, to

107

date, cataracts have rarely been reported in humans, and many psychiatrists do not routinely order eye examinations.

Similarly, there were early fears that *ziprasidone*, which modestly prolongs the QT interval, might lead to torsades de pointes, but again this has not been reported commonly in patients. An additional concern with the newer agents is their high cost. However, this may be balanced by better patient compliance, with lower overall morbidity, leading to fewer hospital days, improved personal relationships, and a greater chance of maintaining employment. The issue of marked weight gain and an increased risk of diabetes with all of the SGAs, with the possible exception of *ziprasidone*, has led the FDA to require the manufacturers of all the second-generation antipsychotics to issue a warning concerning these risks in their product information. Their favorable side effect profiles have led some clinicians to use them as the first choice for antipsychotic therapy and for their adjunctive use in mood stabilization.

Figure 16-2 lists the usual starting doses of the second-generation antipsychotics and their common dosage ranges.

Drug	Usual starting dose	Common dose range
Clozapine	25-50mg PO bid	150-400mg/d
Risperidone	.5-1mg PO bid	2-8mg/d
Olanzapine	7.5-10mg PO hs	10-30mg hs
Quetiapine	25-50mg PO bid	300-500mg/d
Ziprasidone	20-40mg PO bid	40-80mg bid
Aripiprazole	10mg PO qam	15-30mg qam
Lurasidone	20mg PO qd	80-160mg qd
Asenapine	5mg SL bid	5-10mg SL bid
Paliperidone	6mg PO qd	6-12mg PO qd
Iloperidone	1mg PO bid	6-12mg PO bid
Brexpiprazole	1mg PO qd	2-4mg PO qd

Fig. 16-2.   Second-generation antipsychotics.

Figure 16-3 lists the equivalent dosages for some of the older antipsychotic medications (first generation) and the usual therapeutic dosage range.

Drug	Equivalent (oral) dose	Daily therapeutic dosage range for schizophrenia (approx.)
Chlorpromazine	100 mg	200-1600 mg
Perphenazine	8 mg	16-64 mg
Trifluoperazine	5 mg	10-80 mg
Fluphenazine	2 mg	5-40 mg
Thiothixene	5 mg	10-80 mg
Haloperidol	2 mg	5-40 mg

Fig. 16-3.   First-generation antipsychotics.

Side Effects of Antipsychotic Drugs

The major side effects of the older antipsychotic drugs include extrapyramidal reactions and anticholinergic effects. The three major extrapyramidal reactions are the dystonias, akathisia (a movement disorder with a need to be in constant motion), and parkinsonian side effects. Dystonic reactions occur more frequently with older, high potency neuroleptics (e.g., haloperidol), tend to develop early in treatment (first several days), and usually consist of contractions of neck muscles or eye muscles (*oculogyric crisis*). Akathisia is a subjective symptom of extreme inner restlessness and inability to sit still. It tends to develop several days or weeks after instituting therapy. *Pseudoparkinsonism* consists of cogwheel rigidity, pill rolling tremor of the hands, mask-like facial expression, and shuffling gait, which occur 1 to several weeks after starting treatment and are more common with high potency neuroleptics. Anticholinergic side effects include dry mouth, blurred vision, urinary retention, constipation, dry skin and mucous membranes, delirium, and acute glaucoma. Rarely, the *central anticholinergic syndrome* may occur, in which the patient becomes delirious and experiences severe (and life-threatening) autonomic instability. It may seem paradoxical, but anticholinergic drugs are used to treat the extrapyramidal symptoms. *Physostigmine,* an acetylcholinesterase inhibitor, can be used to counteract anticholinergic poisoning.

Tardive dyskinesia is an uncommon extrapyramidal side effect of antipsychotic drugs. It usually consists of spontaneous movements of the face, including rolling the tongue, smacking the lips, and chewing or blowing motions. Less commonly, movements of the trunk or limbs resembling chorea or tics occur. The disorder may begin after only a few months on these medications but more often occurs after several years at relatively high doses. It may be an irreversible side effect.

Other side effects of the neuroleptics include jaundice, leukopenia, pigmentary retinopathy (with thioridazine), and pigment deposits in the skin and the lens of the eye.

All antipsychotic agents, have an FDA "black box warning" for an increased risk of death in elderly patients with dementia-related psychosis. All antipsychotic agents that have an FDA indication for treating bipolar depression (*quetiapine, lurasidone, olanzapine/fluoxetine*) also have the FDA warning regarding the risk of suicidality in children, adolescents, and young adults.

For the emergency treatment of acute psychotic conditions, *haloperidol* is still widely used, but *ziprasidone* IM and *olanzapine* IM have become more common.

Mood Stabilizers

Mood stabilizers are now widely used in psychiatry. The FDA approved *lithium* for the treatment of mania in 1970. In the past 10–15 years the diagnosis of bipolar disorder has become more common. The incidence of classic bipolar I disorder has not changed significantly, but bipolar II and unspecified bipolar disorder have been diagnosed with greater frequency. Some authors write of the "bipolar spectrum" and some include patients with borderline personality and other volatile personality traits.

Since the early 1990's several anticonvulsants and second-generation antipsychotic agents have been approved by the FDA for bipolar disease. *Divalproex* was the first anticonvulsant approved by the FDA, in the mid 1990s, for the treatment of bipolar disorder. *Carbamazepine* was used as an alternative to lithium beginning in the 1970s but not approved by the FDA for this indication until 2004. *Olanzapine* (Zyprexa) was approved for the treatment of mania, and later, in combination with *fluoxetine* (Symbyax), for bipolar depression. *Lamotrigine* (Lamictal) was approved for the maintenance phase of bipolar disorder, and may have particular effectiveness in preventing the recurrence of the depressive phase of the illness. *Risperidone, quetiapine, ziprasidone, and asenapine* have also received indications specifically for use in the manic phase of illness. *Quetiapine* and *lurasidone* have been approved for the depressive phase of bipolar illness.

The newer agents have been increasingly prescribed, but lithium is still considered by many to be the drug of choice for maintenance in patients with classical bipolar I, euphoric manic episodes and severe depressive episodes without comorbid substance abuse. There is also evidence that lithium may make suicide less likely in bipolar patients, who have, overall, a greater than 15% lifetime risk of suicide.

Lithium is effective in the treatment of the manic phase of illness and is secondarily useful in the prevention of manic episodes. To a lesser degree it may prevent depressive episodes. The usual effective dosage range of lithium carbonate is 600–2400mg daily. The actual monitoring of the effective dose is done by checking blood levels, which usually should range from 0.8 to 1.2 meq/L. The exact mechanism by which lithium works is unknown. In patients who are acutely manic, the therapeutic effect of lithium is not observed for at least 1 week, and during that time the use of antipsychotic drugs for behavioral control may be necessary, as well as lithium levels up to 1.5 meq/L.

The side effects of lithium include gastrointestinal symptoms such as nausea, vomiting, diarrhea, and indigestion. These can occur at therapeutic blood levels. Dividing doses helps alleviate these symptoms. Toxic effects of lithium include tremors, ataxia, nystagmus, stupor, and coma. These symptoms usually occur at blood levels over 1.5 meq/L but in some patients may occur at blood levels significantly less than this. Lithium may also cause cardiac arrhythmias. Increased thirst and polyuria are extremely common side effects of lithium treatment. Long-term use of lithium has been associated with decreased urine concentrating ability and hypothyroidism. When considering patients for long-term lithium use, periodic evaluations of kidney and thyroid function should be performed.

Treatment of acute mania with *divalproex* is usually started with a minimum daily dose of 1000mg and rapidly increased to 2000mg per day or higher. The target blood level, measured as valproic acid, is 50–125 micrograms/ml (the upper limit of the range in seizure patients is 100). Side effects include sedation, weight gain, hair loss, and fatigue. Life-threatening liver dysfunction or pancreatitis are very rare but important to remember. Blood dyscrasias (especially granulocytopenia and thrombocytopenia), have been reported. Monitoring includes baseline liver function tests and CBC followed by repeats of these tests plus valproic acid levels at appropriate intervals based on acuity of manic symptoms, usually at one month, then 3–6 month intervals. The *polycystic ovary syndrome* has been associated with the use of valproic acid and divalproex in patients with epilepsy. The risk in bipolar patients is unclear, but concomitant weight gain may be the key risk factor. These agents have also been associated with neural tube defects in infants whose mothers became pregnant while taking the medication, so effective birth control should be advised for all women of child-bearing age while using these drugs. While divalproex is not yet approved for bipolar maintenance, it is commonly used for this indication, with or without lithium or a second generation antipsychotic.

Olanzapine or other second-generation antipsychotics are often added to the medication regimen in acute mania to control symptoms more rapidly, as an alternative to haloperidol, which was used for this purpose for many years. However, the side effect profile of the newer antipsychotics requires close monitoring to ensure that the added burden of diabetes is not induced iatrogenically. *Aripiprazole* has significant antidepressant effects in some patients and is approved by the FDA for adjunctive use with antidepressants in major depression. Other second-generation antipsychotics are occasionally used for this indication as well; their sedative and anxiolytic effects make them particularly useful in patients with treatment-refractory agitated depressions.

Lamotrigine became an important drug in the treatment of bipolar disease for several reasons. As noted, it is particularly useful in the depressive phase of the illness, which comprises 60–70% of the time bipolar patients spend in a mood episode. Patients often report more energy and clearer thinking. And, it has few serious side effects, no weight gain, no sexual side effects, no sedation or impairment of concentration, and few GI effects. Dizziness and diplopia, anxiety, irritability, headaches, or insomnia occasionally occur but are usually transient. The only serious side effect is a 1/1200 risk of developing the *Stevens-Johnson syndrome*. This risk estimate derives from the early use of *lamotrigine* in seizure disorders and the fairly rapid titration schedule that was used at first. With the current titration schedule, 25mg each a.m. for 14 days, 50mg a.m. for the next 14 days, 100mg a.m. for 7 days, and then 200mg daily (patients on *divalproex* start at the above rate due to its enzyme inhibition; those on carbamazepine begin at twice the rate due to its enzyme induction effects), the risk of a serious rash is minimized by careful patient education, close monitoring, and by discontinuation of the drug if a rash occurs.

The long acting intramuscular of risperidone may prove useful for a select group of bipolar patients who might benefit from long-term injectable medication, though it is not approved for this indication at present.

Other medications have been, and continue to be, prescribed in bipolar illness, but clear efficacy in controlled trials has not been demonstrated. *Oxcarbazepine* (Trileptal), a close chemical relative of carbamazepine is now occasionally used, though there are no definitive studies to support its use. *Gabapentin* (Neurontin) was formerly thought to show promise for having significant benefit without significant side effects, but this has not proven true and it is not commonly used. *Topiramate* (Topamax) and *zonesimide* (Zonegran) are other anticonvulsants that have been proposed as adjunctive agents in this illness. *Topiramate* and *zonesimide* have side effects of sedation and weight loss and, especially for *topiramate*, there is anecdotal evidence that these agents may be useful in patients with "bipolar spectrum" characteristics for whom weight gain is a major concern.

Sedative-Hypnotics; Antianxiety Agents

The sedative-hypnotics as a group are often called antianxiety drugs or minor tranquilizers. The *barbiturates* were the first, followed by *meprobamate* (Equanil), *hydroxyzine* (Atarax), and *chlordiazepoxide* (Librium). The *benzodiazepines*, of which *chlordiazepoxide* (Librium) was the first, are by far the most widely used drugs of this class at present. The utility of these drugs lies primarily in the treatment of short-term circumscribed anxiety and insomnia, using the lowest effective dose for the shortest period of time possible. Practically speaking, this means the use of *lorazepam* (Ativan) 1mg tid (or the equivalent dose of another benzodiazepine) or less for no more than 2–3 weeks. Of course, these drugs are also useful in the treatment of alcohol withdrawal.

Alprazolam (Xanax) has an FDA indication for use in panic disorder. However, many patients rapidly develop a tolerance to *alprazolam* and other benzodiazepines. There is a fine line between the clear potential for abuse of drugs in this class and their effectiveness for certain symptoms. Other commonly used benzodiazepines include *clonazepam* (Klonopin), which is indicated for seizures but is also used for panic. *Clonazepam* has a slower onset of action and a longer half-life than *alprazolam,* and while some clinicians believe it has less potential for addiction, this is not the case. *Oxazepam* (Serax) is occasionally used for alcohol withdrawal and *clorazepate* (Tranxene) is used for anxiety. Benzodiazepines significantly add to the risk of unintentional overdoses in patients who also use opioids for pain.

Generalized anxiety disorder is now most often treated by psychiatrists with SSRIs and SNRIs, such as *paroxetine, sertraline, venlafaxine,* or *escitalopram,* as noted above. However, *buspirone* may be helpful.

Buspirone (Buspar) is unrelated to the benzodiazepines and is not addictive. Many patients who have previously taken a benzodiazepine complain that *buspirone* is ineffective. In fact, it can be quite useful in certain patients, but its onset of action is similar to the antidepressants, 2–6 weeks, so the patient must be reassured. The usual starting dose is 7.5mg bid; the dose is then titrated upward to 15–30mg bid. Common side effects are dizziness and nausea, which usually disappear within a few weeks.

Zolpidem (Ambien) is one of the most commonly used sedatives today. It is a non-benzodiazepine gamma-aminobutyric acid (GABA) agonist. Related sedatives include *eszopiclone* (Lunesta) and *zaleplon.* Each of these agents has a rapid onset of action and usually little residual morning drowsiness. Tolerance develops to them, so brief or intermittent use is indicated. They share side effects with the benzodiazepines. Anterograde amnesia is a potentially serious side effect of these agents as well as of high potency short-acting benzodiazepines such as *triazolam*. Use of alcohol increases the risk.

Ramelteon (Rozerem) is a melatonin receptor agonist that has FDA approval for insomnia. It is unrelated to the other sedatives and has no apparent potential for development of dependence.

Adjunctive Medications for Alcohol Treatment

Disulfiram (Antabuse) is a drug that can be an effective adjunct in the treatment of alcohol use disorders. Patients who drink alcohol after having taken this drug will have an alcohol-Antabuse reaction. The reaction consists of skin flushing, elevated pulse rate, increased respiration, hypotension, chest pain, nausea, copious vomiting, diaphoresis, and blurred vision. Severe reactions may lead to respiratory depression, cardiovascular collapse, cardiac arrhythmias, congestive heart failure, seizures, and death. The drug is therefore useful only in those patients who sincerely wish to stop drinking and may be likely to drink on impulse. The usual dose range is 250-500mg daily. The drug is only an adjunct to a comprehensive alcohol treatment approach as outlined in Chapter 8.

Naltrexone (Revia and others), an opiate antagonist/agonist, was originally developed for the treatment of opiate dependence. It was approved by the FDA to aid in the treatment of alcohol dependence. Studies have shown that *naltrexone* reduces the craving for alcohol in some patients and may reduce the euphoric effects of alcohol, leading to decreased consumption of alcohol when a patient does drink. The usual dose is 50mg HS, although some studies have shown higher doses (75-100mg hs) to be more effective. As with *disulfiram, naltrexone* is only an adjunctive agent. *Acamprosate* (Campral) has also received an FDA indication for use in the treatment of alcohol use disorders and has potential benefits similar to *naltrexone*, although certain patients may find one or the other to be significantly more efficacious. The effective dose of *acamprosate* is 666mg tid.

Other drugs have been studied for use in alcohol treatment. Positive studies have been published for benefits with alcohol craving, and reductions in alcohol use, with *topiramate* (Topamax), an anticonvulsant, and *ondansetron* (Zofran), an anti-nausea medication used in chemotherapy patients. *Gabapentin* has been used in alcohol withdrawal protocols as well in an attempt to reduce anxiety and craving in patients who are trying to reduce their alcohol intake.

Electroconvulsive Therapy

Electroconvulsive therapy (ECT) is the most maligned treatment modality in psychiatry. It consists of strategically placing electrodes on the scalp (either in the temporal region bilaterally or 1 electrode at the vertex of the scalp and the other at the temporal region on the non-dominant side). Then, a precisely measured electrical impulse is passed through the brain. This causes a generalized convulsive seizure. Pretreatment with a short-acting barbiturate, such as sodium thiopental, and a short-acting muscle relaxant, such as succinylcholine, is necessary. This allows the patient to experience only a very short-term general anesthesia and a significant diminution of the tonic-clonic movements in the generalized seizure. Therapeutic response is correlated with total seizure time.

Following the treatment, the patient is postictal, confused, and disoriented to time, and sometimes place. The patient may have a headache and some muscular pains. These symptoms last only a few hours. The most troublesome side effect is short-term memory loss, which lasts several hours to several days. Rarely, patients will complain of long-term memory problems. The use of unilateral ECT with the electrical current passing through the non-dominant hemisphere reduces the degree of memory loss. The efficacy of ECT in severe depression is considerable, with 80% or more of patients with severe depressions having a markedly positive response. ECT is mainly used in patients who have not responded to adequate trials of several antidepressants, patients who have had a positive response to ECT in the past, or patients who are in life-threatening situations. For example, patients who are imminently suicidal (and depressed) or severely catatonic (and not eating or drinking) may not be able to wait for medications to take effect.

Transcranial Magnetic Stimulation

Repetitive *transcranial magnetic stimulation (rTMS)* uses magnetic coils applied to the head to produce a magnetic field in the brain and stimulate nerve cells. It was approved by the FDA for the treatment of depression and is used primarily in treatment-resistant cases. The treatment involves 45-50 minutes sessions 4 or 5 days a week for a total of approximately 20 treatments. TMS is not as effective as ECT in patients with severe depression but may be helpful to certain patients.

Deep Brain Stimulation

Deep brain stimulation (DBS) is a neurosurgical procedure in which electrodes are placed in certain brain regions and stimulated with a pacemaker device. The only psychiatric indication approved by the FDA for DBS is obsessive-compulsive disorder, but it has been studied for the treatment of severe recurrent depressions and may be effective in selected cases. DBS has been approved by the FDA for neurological conditions, including Parkinson's Disease.

Exercise

Recommending exercise is considered "common sense" by many patients, but some clinicians are unaware that there are a number of research studies including several randomized controlled trials (RCTs) that show 'its efficacy in the treatment of major depression. Several studies by Madhukar Trivedi at the University of Texas Southwestern Medical Center as well as researchers at other clinics have confirmed that the "exercise dose" recommended by US guidelines ("2008 Physical Activity Guidelines for Americans") is effective in the treatment of mild to moderate major depression. This dose is defined as 150 minutes of mild-moderate intensity or 75 minutes of vigorous aerobic exercise each week, or a combination. *Mild to moderate* is defined as brisk walking (3 miles/hour or faster), and *vigorous* is defined as running, jogging, swimming laps, or the equivalent in other forms of exercise.

CLINICAL REVIEW

It's time to test your knowledge of psychiatry. We hope that the previous chapters have made this specialty more comprehensible! Here we go.

(1) Question:
A 25-year-old woman complains of lower back pain. She also appears depressed. How should you evaluate her?
A) Ask her about other symptoms of depression.
B) Evaluate her back pain; ignore the depression.
C) Evaluate her depression; ignore the back pain.
D) Refer her to a psychiatrist.
Answer: A. Other symptoms of depression include the vegetative signs and suicidal ideation. Her back pain should be seriously evaluated. It could be a depressive equivalent or another medical problem. A referral to a psychiatrist might be appropriate. However, if she is suicidal, it's not safe to let her out of your office until a disposition is arranged. Remember, many people who suicide have seen their primary care physician in the preceding several weeks.

(2) Question:
The patient has been depressed for 4 months but not suicidal, and you learn her mother died around the onset of her depressive symptoms. Should you refer her to a psychiatrist?
Answer: Not necessarily. Many patients prefer treatment from their primary care physician. They are reluctant to accept a psychiatric referral or diagnosis. Grief does not preclude the diagnosis of depression (DSM-5) if other depressive symptoms meet the diagnostic criteria.

(3) Question:
Should you start this woman on antidepressant medication?
Answer: Probably, if supportive care is ineffective. Make sure she is not allergic to the antidepressant you choose. Pregnancy generally precludes the use of antidepressants, but in some cases of severe depression they may be considered with

care, coordinated with the obstetrician and a psychiatrist. For example, begin with 25mg of *sertraline* for 4–6 days, and then increase to 50mg. If there is no response after 4 weeks, increase to 100mg. Alternatively, begin with a daily dose of 10mg of *fluoxetine* for 4-6 days, then increase to 20mg daily. If there is no response after 4 weeks, increase to 40mg. The lethality of SSRI antidepressants in overdose is relatively low. However, it is prudent to prescribe all psychotropic medications cautiously. Depressed outpatients should initially be seen several times a month to monitor their symptoms.

(4) Question:
Ten days later, the patient is still depressed. What should your next action be?
A) Change medication.
B) Stop medication.
C) Continue medication.
D) Recommend ECT.
Answer: C. Antidepressants begin to relieve symptoms of depression after 2–4 weeks. Continue medicating the patient. If there is a partial response, maximize the dose or augment with another antidepressant. If treatment fails, change to another antidepressant in a different class.

(5) Question:
The patient is better. How long should you continue her antidepressants?
Answer: In a patient with a single episode of depression, continue the medication for a minimum of 6-9 months. Then taper the antidepressant slowly, e.g., reduce the daily dose by 25% every 2-4 weeks and then discontinue. This is necessary because some patients develop withdrawal symptoms (nausea, insomnia, irritability). Follow the patient monthly, or every other month, for 6 more months. For patients with recurrent depressive episodes, ongoing antidepressant treatment is usually necessary.

(6) Question:
A 35-year-old severely depressed woman has been hospitalized with suicidal ideation and on antidepressant medication for 10 days. She suddenly becomes more pleasant, more organized, pays her 2-month-old doctor's bill, and arranges her affairs at home through a relative who is living there. She comes to you and asks to be discharged from the hospital. Should you let her go?
Answer: Probably not. When depressed patients appear brighter, happier, more organized, and in charge of their affairs, these can be signs that they have secretly decided to commit suicide. You would want to do a very careful suicide evaluation and observe the patient before making any decision to let her leave the hospital. Of course, your treatment may be working, but antidepressants usually take 2-4 weeks to take effect, and the full effect of a given dose of medication may not be clear for 8 weeks or more. Suicide is more common early in treatment, when patients have increased energy from the medication but still feel and think their situation is hopeless.

(7) Question:

A 22-year-old woman has had symptoms of anxiety and depression intermittently for the last 5 years. After 1 year of psychotherapy, she develops a transient paralysis of her left arm the morning after taking a sleeping pill. What is your differential diagnosis?

Answer: She could have acute intermittent porphyria, which causes psychological symptoms, neuropathies, and abdominal pain. Porphyria often follows ingestion of barbiturate. She could have a conversion disorder, and this would be corroborated by the psychological findings of previous history of conversion symptoms, identifying with a relative who had a similar symptom, and an immediate (recent) psychological stressor. She also could have both a psychiatric condition and a neurologic condition.

(8) Question:

A 20-year-old man is angry at his college professor for giving him a weekend assignment. Shortly after growing angry, he faints. What's wrong with him?

Answer:

He could have suffered a conversion symptom. He also could have narcolepsy. Remember, in this disorder, cataplexy (loss of motor tone in response to a strong emotion), may be accompanied by hypnogogic hallucinations, sleep paralysis, and daytime drowsiness.

(9) Question:

A 39-year-old woman complains of fatigue and trouble falling asleep. What should you do to evaluate her?

Answer:

Do a history, physical exam, and mental status exam. Remember ABSTRACT and DEEP.

(10) Question:

The mental status exam on this patient shows auditory hallucinations, disorientation, and memory impairment. What is the most likely diagnosis?

A) Schizophrenia.

B) Delirium or Dementia.

C) Depression.

D) Narcolepsy.

Answer:

The answer is B. Delirium is characterized by disorientation, and memory impairment is a key feature of dementia. Hallucinations and delusions can also occur in a delirium.

(11) Question:

A workup for physiologic causes of the patient's symptoms is negative. Could she have a psychiatric illness?

Answer:
Yes. Sometimes depression causes disorientation and memory impairment. This is termed *pseudodementia.*

(12) Question:
How many psychiatrists does it take to change a light bulb?
Answer:
It only takes one, but the light bulb has to want to change. On the surface, this seems a simple joke. In fact, it really is hard to get patients to change their behavior or alter their symptoms if they aren't willing to participate in the treatment themselves.

(13) Question:
A 22-year-old schizophrenic patient is admitted with a worsening of his psychotic symptoms and tardive dyskinesia. What is your differential diagnosis?
Answer: He probably has schizophrenia and a tardive dyskinesia. Tardive dyskinesias are late sequelae of neuroleptic treatment. They are motor movements (usually about the mouth and face) that are often irreversible. He also could have Huntington's chorea. Remember, in this illness, schizophrenia-like symptoms can precede the development of the choreiform movements. Wilson's disease causes mental status changes and extrapyramidal signs and symptoms. Don't assume that a patient who appears schizophrenic has schizophrenia. The differential diagnosis is important.

(14) Question:
A 65-year-old businessman develops auditory hallucinations, paranoia, and anxiety. What is the most likely diagnosis?
A) Schizophrenia.
B) Bipolar Disorder.
C) Neurocognitive disorder.
D) Sleep apnea.
Answer: C. Schizophrenia usually begins before age 45. Bipolar disorder can start late in life. However, the primary problem is an altered mood. Delirium involves disorientation; memory impairment denotes dementia; and psychotic symptoms (hallucinations, paranoia) may accompany either. These symptoms, at this age, will lead the clinician to place Frontotemporal Neurocognitive Disorder and Neurocognitive Disorder with Lewy Bodies at the top of the differential diagnoses (DSM-5).

(15) Question:
In which condition(s) is the risk for suicide increased?
A) Depression.
B) Alcoholism.
C) Anorexia Nervosa.
D) Schizophrenia.
Answer: The suicide risk is increased in all these conditions. Remember SUICIDAL.

(16) Question:
A 14-year-old girl lost 30 pounds and now weighs 80 pounds. Medical history, physical exam, and laboratory tests, including electrolytes, are normal. How best do you proceed?
A) Diagnose anorexia nervosa and refer her to a psychiatrist.
B) Tell her she needs to gain weight.
C) No intervention is necessary.
D) Diagnose anorexia nervosa and treat her yourself.
Answer: B. Remember **LOW** FOOD. This patient has *L*oss *of* *W*eight. Look for *F*ear *Of O*besity, *Distortion of body image*. Tell her she needs to gain weight and see if she complies. If she *Refuses* to try to gain weight, it's diagnostic of anorexia nervosa.

(17) Question:
The patient refuses to eat. What should you do next?
A) Refer her to a psychiatrist.
B) Treat her yourself.
C) Have her sign an AMA (against medical advice) form.
D) Threaten her with hospitalization.
Answer: A. Psychiatrists should help treat these patients.

(18) Question:
What is the differential diagnosis of enuresis?
Answer: CAP'IM! CNS, anatomical, psychological, infectious, and metabolic problems can cause enuresis.

(19) Question:
How do you evaluate a 7-year-old enuretic boy?
Answer: Look for psychological causes (anger, ambition). Check a urinalysis (to rule out juvenile onset diabetes mellitus, urinary tract infection, and kidney disease). Do not perform an invasive procedure (e.g., cystoscopy) until other causes are excluded.

(20) Question:
Should a 7-year-old fire-setter be referred to a child psychiatrist?
Answer: Yes! Fire-setting is serious antisocial behavior. Psychiatric treatment is necessary.

(21) Question:
Is somnambulism (sleep walking) safe?
Answer: No. Make sure the somnambulist's room has locked windows and no obstacles.

(22) Question:
What condition(s) can be treated with imipramine?
A) Enuresis.
B) Depression.

C) Seizures.
D) Encopresis (soiling).
Answer: A and B. Tricyclic antidepressants have anticholinergic properties. Bladder capacity increases; enuresis usually stops. These antidepressants also, of course, treat depression.

(23) Question:
What condition(s) can be treated with amphetamines?
A) Attention-Deficit/Hyperactivity Disorder.
B) Depression.
C) Obesity.
D) Narcolepsy.
Answer: A, B, and D. Amphetamines transiently elevate mood. They may work in treatment-resistant depression, particularly in the elderly. Anorexia is a side effect of amphetamines. However, their use in treating obesity is dangerous.

(24) Question:
A 22-year-old man develops a delusion. He believes that Jimmy Fallon wants him to be a guest host on the Tonight Show. How would you characterize this delusion?
A) Paranoid.
B) Gradiose.
C) Realistic.
D) Somatic.
Answer: B.

(25) Question:
What is the most likely diagnosis for this man?
Answer: Schizophrenia. Other symptoms of schizophrenia are hallucinations, catatonia, and disorganized thinking!

(26) Question:
A 20-year-old man believes that the FBI wants to hurt him. What kind of delusion is this?
Answer: Paranoid.

(27) Question:
The same 20-year-old man denies hallucinations. What is the most likely diagnosis in his case?
Answer: Delusional disorder. Delusions without accompanying hallucinations, catatonia, disorganized thinking, or the "negative symptoms" of schizophrenia is delusional disorder!

(28) Question:
Which of the following statements is most true about Sigmund Freud?
A) He was a famous baseball player for the New York Mets.
B) He conducts a famous symphony.

C) He was a neurologist.

D) He writes the gourmet section for a famous newspaper.

Answer: C. He was a neurologist. Is that surprising? Modern psychiatry and psychoanalysis actually were an outgrowth of neurology. In the 20th century, psychiatry became a separate specialty, but now it appears to be moving closer to neurology and the "medical" sciences.

(29) Question:

A 40-year-old man with chronic schizophrenia has had a fixed delusion that the telephone wires are talking to him for the past 15 years. He has also heard voices commenting on his behavior for 10 years. In the last month, he has developed visual hallucinations of spiders crawling down his wall. He now believes the television is talking to him. Why have his symptoms changed?

Answer: Psychotic symptoms tend to remain stable over time. If a schizophrenic patient has a change of symptoms, suspect the possibility that another condition is causing the new psychotic symptoms. He could have a delirium or dementia (he has visual hallucinations now), a brain tumor, or a worsening of the schizophrenic condition.

(30) Question:

A 35-year-old woman with chronic schizophrenia was readmitted to the state hospital with an exacerbation of her chronic paranoid symptoms. She briefly mentioned complaints of occasionally seeing snakes and difficulty concentrating. Her doctor increased her antipsychotic meds, but her symptoms persisted. What's missing here?

Answer: ABSTRACT—Review of patient's records revealed that Cognitive function was normal one year previously and Thought content had contained no hallucinations of snakes. On testing of Attention, serial 7''s and digit span were done poorly; and memory was impaired (2/4 objects/5 min). The patient was referred to a neurologist, who suggested a CT scan. The scan revealed a large temporal lobe tumor. Key points: Always do a mental status examination! Change in symptom patterns and new deficits on mental status examinations suggest organic impairment.

(31) Question:

A 25-year-old woman develops a delusion that she runs the world. Mental status exam reveals no hallucinations, loose associations, or cognitive impairment. What is her most likely diagnosis?

Answer: Bipolar Disorder (manic phase). *Grandiose* delusions accompany manic-depressive illness. A mood disturbance (euphoria or depression) is usually prominent. However, grandiosity can precede the mood change.

(32) Question:

The next day, her mood is very elevated. How should you treat her?

A) Lithium, or other mood stabilizer, as an outpatient.

B) Lithium, or other mood stabilizer, as an inpatient.

C) Antidepressants.
D) ECT.
Answer: B. Bipolar patients can become psychotic and agitated quickly. It is best to admit these patients if possible. Mood stabilizers, such as *lithium* and *divalproex* are the treatment of choice for bipolar mania. They take 1-2 weeks to reduce manic symptoms. Antipsychotics, also used as mood stabilizers (e.g., *olanzapine, quetiapine,* or *haloperidol*) are also effective. They work in 2–3 days but have more serious side effects (e.g., tardive dyskinesia, diabetes). They are often used until the initial mood stabilizer takes effect.

(33) Question:
A 55-year-old man insists he has cancer of the bowel. A medical workup does not substantiate his concern. The rest of his mental status exam is normal. What is his most likely diagnosis?
A) Delirium/Dementia
B) Conversion Disorder.
C) Paranoia.
D) Depression.
Answer: D. Depression can cause *somatic* delusions. Conversion disorders cause loss or alteration of neurologic functioning. Paranoia causes paranoid delusions. Dementia involves memory impairment, and disorientation accompanies delirium.

(34) Question:
A middle-aged man was rushed to a hospital where he had a cardiac arrest. The EKG returned to normal several hours after resuscitation. Coronary angiography and treadmill EKG were normal. The patient gave a history of spontaneous episodes of hyperventilation, tachycardia with fear, and sweating, all occurring several times per week. Was this a yogi who had developed control of his autonomic nervous system to the point that he could stop his heart?
Answer: No. This is a patient with panic disorder (anxiety attacks). Arrhythmias can cause panic attacks. Don't tell these patients "It's all in your head." Many can benefit from SSRIs or SNRIs. MAO inhibitors are very helpful for patients with panic disorder but are less commonly used today. Benzodiazepines such as lorazepam or alprazolam may reduce panic symptoms when taken at the onset of a panic attack, but the risk of dependence is significant, so they should be used cautiously. The patient should be referred to a psychiatrist and, of course, continue with a cardiologist for further evaluation.

(35) Question:
The patient is a well-dressed 40-year-old woman whom you have been treating for manic-depressive illness with lithium. When she arrives for her monthly medication follow-up at 9:00 a.m., you wonder if you smell alcohol on her breath. You fear offending the patient with a question regarding alcohol use. What should you do?
Answer: Ask directly, with a concerned rather than confrontational tone, "Have you had a drink this morning?" She may be relieved to share her concern over

her problem and ask for help. Remember, alcoholism is common in patients with affective disorders.

(36) Question:
A 46-year-old reserved and conservative businessman suffers a personality change over the course of 6 months. He becomes garrulous, spends a lot of money, and has several sexual affairs. What is your differential diagnosis?
Answer: The first illness to consider is *bipolar disorder*. It can present at this age and manifests with grandiosity and elevated mood. He could be abusing drugs. Cocaine causes grandiosity, hypersexuality, and similar symptoms. Next, brain tumors can cause personality changes. Last, he could be having a mid-life crisis.

(37) Question:
Which mental illness has the best prognosis?
A) Schizophrenia.
B) Bipolar Disorder.
C) Delusional Disorder.
Answer: B. Between episodes, as many as 50% of bipolar patients function well (e.g., have families and jobs). Usually, schizophrenia and delusional disorder are more chronic and debilitating illnesses.

(38) Question:
How should you treat a 40-year-old *alprazolam* (Xanax) addict?
A) Hospitalize and immediately stop all medications.
B) Hospitalize and wean him from his Xanax.
C) Gradually reduce his Xanax. No need to hospitalize.
D) Start him on methadone.
Answer: B or C. Abrupt sedative withdrawal can cause tachycardia, hypertension, delirium, and seizures. The best treatment for patients with dependence on high doses of sedatives is hospitalization to taper the dose of the sedative; however, some motivated, responsible patients may succeed with outpatient withdrawal from more moderate doses (e.g., 3-4mg daily dose).

(39) Question:
What causes Kayser-Fleischer rings?
Answer: Wilson's disease. These are copper deposits in the cornea.

(40) Question:
Why should a psychiatrist know this?
Answer: Wilson's disease also causes psychiatric symptoms.

(41) Question:
A 30-year-old schizophrenic is started on *risperidone*. He develops torticollis (an extrapyramidal side-effect of antipsychotics). *Benztropine* (anticholinergic)

is used to treat this symptom. Two days later, he develops a fever, tachycardia, blurred vision, and visual hallucinations. How should you treat him?
A) Stop the *risperidone* and *benztropine*
B) Give him more *benztropine*
C) Give him more *risperidone*.
D) Give him *diazepam*
Answer: A. He has anticholinergic symptoms. These include dry mouth, blurred vision, elevated temperature, and delirium. The medications that have anticholinergic properties *(benztropine)* should be stopped . It is also important to consider the neuroleptic malignant syndrome, which is treated with supportive care and by withholding antipsychotics, in conjunction with a neurologist.

(42) Question:
A 30-year-old schizophrenic man is medicated with *haloperidol*, 30mg per day. On the 10th day of treatment, he becomes catatonic. What should you do?
A) Increase his *haloperidol*.
B) Administer ECT.
C) Decrease his *haloperidol*.
D) Make no changes in his treatment.
Answer: C. Antipsychotics occasionally cause catatonia. When a patient is medicated with an antipsychotic and develops catatonia, the medication should be stopped. This is a diagnostic maneuver. If the catatonia stops, it probably is due to the antipsychotic, *haloperidol*.

(43) Question:
How do antipsychotic medications work?
A) They are dopamine agonists.
B) They are dopamine antagonists.
C) They block the reuptake of catacholamines.
D) They have anticholinergic properties.
Answer: B. Antipsychotic medications have dopamine antagonist activity. Some have serotonergic activity and some have anticholinergic properties.

(44) Question:
A 25-year-old man is admitted with a 3-week history of auditory hallucinations, delusions, and confusion. He has no previous history of a mental disorder. What diagnoses are consistent with this clinical presentation?
A) Amphetamine-induced psychotic disorder.
B) Brief psychotic disorder.
C) Schizophrenia.
D) Generalized anxiety.
Answer: A and B. Remember, amphetamines can cause psychosis. *Brief psychotic disorder* is diagnosed when disorganized or psychotic symptoms have been present at least 1 day but less than 1 month. It has a much better prognosis than schizophrenia. Schizophrenia is not consistent with this presentation as the patient

must have symptoms of schizophrenia for at least 6 months to meet criteria for the diagnosis.

(45) Question:
What should you do first for this man?
(A) Medicate with an antipsychotic.
(B) Medicate with a sedative (e.g., *lorazepam*).
(C) History and physical exam.
(D) Seclude.
Answer: C. Do a history and physical. Look for signs of amphetamine ingestion (dilated pupils, elevated vital signs). Seclude only if the patient is an imminent danger to himself or others on the unit.

(46) Question:
The history and physical are normal. When would you prescribe an antipsychotic?
Answer: When possible, it's better to wait for a few days. See if the patient calms down on the ward. His hallucinations and delusions may resolve spontaneously. Medicate him sooner if his psychotic symptoms are causing him to be combative, suicidal, or disruptive. Remember, he could have taken other drugs that can cause a psychosis. If he took an anticholinergic drug, don't prescribe antipsychotics. Many agents in this class of drugs have anticholinergic properties.

(47) Question:
A 25-year-old man is caught exposing his genitals to women in a grocery store. Which answer best correlates with a person displaying this behavior?
A) He comes from a low socioeconomic background.
B) He has a history of antisocial behavior and alcohol abuse since his early teens.
C) He has passive-dependent problems. He is making perverted sexual advances, hoping a woman will respond sympathetically and take care of him.
D) He has a defect in neurotransmitter synthesis.
Answer: B. Antisocial behavior, antisocial personality, and alcohol use disorder are risk factors for *exhibitionistic disorder* in males; the disorder is much less common in females.

(48) Question:
What does it mean when people say, "a stitch in time saves nine"?
A) A stitch now will save you a lot of sewing later.
B) A stitch is a twitch that will stretch the material.
C) Don't procrastinate. A little work now can save a lot of work later.
D) My stitches got pulled out by the doctor. He put 10 in, and I won at the horse track.
Answer: C. A is an example of a concrete answer, seen in people who have intellectual trouble with abstractions, or who have a dementia. B shows clanging associations, seen in mania. D shows loose and idiosyncratic associations (disorganized thinking).

(49) Question:

A 30-year-old depressed man complains that he does not ejaculate with orgasm. Is this a delusion?

Answer: No. Some many common antidepressant medications (especially SSRIs and SNRIs) sometimes cause delayed ejaculation or even anorgasmia. Explain this possible side effect to patients before prescribing the medicine.

(50) Question:

A 20-year-old man wants a sex change operation. Which psychiatric condition is occasionally an indication for this surgery?

A) Schizophrenia.

B) Gender dysphoria (DSM-5)

C) Homosexuality with feminine characteristics.

Answer: B. A male with *gender dysphoria* has always felt himself to be a woman. He should have a history of feminine behavior since early childhood. His mental status exam should be normal.

A: Suggested Reading

Kaplan and Sadock's Comprehensive Textbook of Psychiatry, Ninth Edition, Benjamin J Sadock, (ed.), Virginia A Sadock (ed.), and Pedro Ruiz (ed.) (2009)

Essentials of Clinical Psychopharmacology, Third Edition, Alan F Schatzberg (ed.), Charles B Nemeroff (ed.) (2013)

Drugs, Addiction, and the Brain, George F Koob, Michael A Arends, and Michel Le Moal (2014)

Cognitive Behavior Therapy: Basics and Beyond, Second Edition, Judith Beck (2011)

Learning Cognitive-Behavior Therapy: An Illustrated Guide, Jesse Wright, Monica Basco, Michael Thase (2005)

DBT Skills Training Manual, Second Edition, Marsha Linehan (2014)

Interpersonal Psychotherapy of Depression, Gerald Klerman and Myrna Weissman (1994)

Motivational Interviewing: Helping People Change, Third Edition, William R. Miller and Stephen Rollnick (2012)

Handbook of Motivation and Change: A Practical Guide for Clinicians, Petros Levounis and Bachaar Arnaout (2010)

Guided Mindfulness Meditation Jon Kabat-Zinn (2005)

Mindfulness-Based Cognitive Therapy for Depression, Second Edition, Zindel Segal, John Teasdale, and Mark Williams (2012)

Acceptance and Commitment Therapy: The Process and Practice of Mindful Change, Second Edition, Steven Hayes, Kirk Strosahl, and Kelly Wilson (2011)

Eating Disorders: A Guide to Medical Care and Complications, Second Edition, Philip Mehler and Arnold Andersen (2010)

Psychodynamic Psychiatry in Clinical Practice, Fifth Edition, Glen Gabbard (2014)

Psychodynamic Psychotherapy: A Clinical Manual, Deborah Cabaniss (2011)

INDEX

Words in italics refer to terminology changes in the DSM-5 classification.

Abilify, 18, 107
ABSTRACT, 7
acamprosate, 47, 113
Acceptance and Commitment
    Therapy, 97
acetozalamide, 71
acting out, 93
acute brain syndrome, 33
acute intermittent porphyria, 38, 65, 72
Acute Stress Disorder, 41
Adderall, 82
addiction, 44
Addison's disease, 70
ADHD, 79
Adjustment Disorders, 41
advanced phase type sleep disorder, 55
affect, 7
affective flattening, 23
agoraphobia, 36, 37
alcoholism, 44, 45
alexythymia, 7
alogia, 23
alprazolam, 41, 112, 114
altered mental status, 33
aluminum poisoning, 69
Alzheimer's Dementia, 34
Ambien, 112
ambivalence, 24
amitriptyline, 100, 104
amphetamines, 49
anabolic steroids, 50

Anafranil, 105
anhedonia, 23
anorexia nervosa, 57, 62
Antabuse, 113
antianxiety agents, 112
antidepresants, 100
antipsychotic agents, 107
Antisocial Personality Disorder, 77,
    87, 89, 91
anxiety in childhood, 79
anxiety, 36
aripiprazole, 18, 20, 25, 26, 27, 107,
    108, 111
arsenic poisoning, 70
arteriosclerotic brain disease, 34
asenapine, 25, 107, 108, 110
Atarax, 112
atenolol and depression, 71
Ativan, 41, 112
atomoxetine, 82
Attention-Deficit/Hyperactivity
    Disorder (ADHD), 79, 82
atypical antipsychotics, 107
Autism Spectrum Disorder (ASD),
    76, 81
autism, 24, 76
automatic thoughts, 96
Avoidant Personality Disorder, 88
Avoidant Restrictive Food Intake
    Disorder, 57, 60
avolition, 23

baclofen, 42
BAD SHAPE, 87
barbiturates, 49, 112
bath salts, 50
Beck Depression Inventory, 105
benzodiazepines, 49, 112
benztropine, 124
beta blockers and depression, 71
betaxolol, 71
Binge Eating Disorder, 57, 60
bipolar depression, 11
Bipolar Disorder Due to Another Medical Condition, 30
bipolar disorder, 23, 28
Bipolar I Disorder, 30
Bipolar II Disorder, 30
body dysmorphic disorder, 40
Borderline Personality Disorder, 87, 88, 90
Breathing-Related Sleep Disorders, 54
brexpiprazole, 25, 107, 108
Brief Psychotic Disorder, 24, 125
Brintellix, 104
bromide poisoning, 70
bulimia nervosa, 57, 58, 62
buprenorphine, 51
bupropion, 18, 19, 101, 103, 106
Buspar, 112
buspirone, 42, 101, 112

caffeine, 50
Campral, 113
carbamazepine, 31, 110
carcinoid tumors, 38
catastrophic reaction, 38
catatonia, 12, 24
Celexa, 18, 102
central anticholinergic syndrome, 109
Central Sleep Apnea, 54
child abuse, 80
chlordiazepoxide, 112
chlorpromazine, 26, 107, 108, 112
Cialis, 101
cimetidine, 71

Circadian Rhythm Sleep-Wake Disorder, 54
circumstantial thought, 8
citalopram, 18, 19, 101, 102, 106
clanging, 8, 126
classical conditioning, 96
client-centered/gestalt/existential psychotherapy, 95
clinician confidentiality, 5
clinician fidelity, 5
clomipramine, 42, 43, 105
clonazepam, 41, 112
clorazepate, 112
clozapine, 25, 107, 108
Clozaril, 107
Cluster A personality disorders, 88
Cluster B personalty disorders, 88
Cluster C personality disorders, 88
codeine, 48, 49
cognition, 9
cognitive behavior therapy, 18, 31, 91, 95
cognitive model, 3
cognitive processing therapy (CPT), 42
cognitive-behavioral psychotherapy, 95
compulsions, 39
Conduct Disorder, 77
Conversion Disorder, 64, 65, 67
coprolalia, 80
countertransference, 65, 94
crack, 49
crystal meth, 49, 50
Cushing's disease, 70
Cyclothymia, 30
Cymbalta, 18, 103

DBS, 19
deep brain stimulation, 19, 114
DEEP, 53
delayed ejaculation, 83
delayed phase type sleep disorder, 55
delirium tremens (DTs), 34, 46
delirium, 22, 23, 33
delusional (paranoid) disorder, 25
delusional disorder, 22

Dementia with Lewy Bodies, 34
dementia, 22, 23, 33
Dependent Personality Disorder, 87
depersonalization, 41, 89
depersonalization/derealization
   disorder, 41
depression in childhood, 79
depression, 11, 64
Depressive Disorder due to another
   medical condition, 13
depressive equivalents, 79
derailment, 8
derealization, 41, 89
desipramine, 100
desvenlafaxine, 18, 19, 103
Desyrel, 104
Dexedrine, 82
dextroamphetamine, 82
Diagnostic and Statistical Manual of
   Mental Disorders, 5th Edition, 1
Dialectical Behavior Therapy, 90, 97, 98
diazepam, 41
diphenhydramine, 56
Disruptive Mood Dysregulation
   Disorder (DMDD), 79
dissociative amnesia, 41
Dissociative Identity Disorder (DID), 41
disulfiram, 47, 113
divalproex, 31, 110
doxepin, 26, 100, 104
doxylamine, 56
DSM-5, 1
DTs (delirium tremens), 46
duloxetine, 18, 19, 103, 106

Eating Disorder NOS (Not Otherwise
   Specified), 57
eating disorders, 57
echolalia, 76
ECT, 19, 106, 113
Effexor, 18, 103
ego-defense mechanisms, 93
ego-dystonic conditions, 87
ego, 93
Elavil, 100

electro-convulsive therapy, 19, 31,
   106, 113
encephalopathy, 33
encopresis, 121
enuresis, 75, 81
Equanil, 112
erectile disorder, 83, 84, 85
Erotomanic Delusional Disorder,
   25
escitalopram, 18, 19, 101, 102, 106
eszopiclone, 55, 112
exhibitionistic disorder, 86, 126
Existential Psychotherapy, 98
Existential-Humanistic Psychotherapy,
   98
eye movement desensitization &
   reprocessing therapy, 42

Factitious Disorder by proxy, 67
Factitious Disorder, 64, 66
Family Systems Therapy, 100
Family Therapy, 100
Fanapt, 107
female orgasmic disorder, 83, 84, 85
female sexual interest/arousal
   disorder, 83, 84
fentanyl, 48
fetishistic disorder, 86
Fetzima, 103
first-generation antipsychotics (FGA),
   26
first-generation antipsychotics, 108
flight of ideas, 8
fluoxetine, 18, 19, 32, 43, 62, 101,
   102, 106, 110, 117
fluphenazine, 107, 108
flurazepam, 56
fluvoxamine, 101
Freud, 92
Freud's structural model, 93
Freud's topological model, 93
Freudian psychoanalysts, 94
Frontotemporal Neurocognitive
   Disorder, 119
frotteuristic disorder, 86

Functional Neurological Symptoms
  Disorder, 64, 65
gabapentin, 42, 47, 111, 113
Gambling Disorder, 50
gamma-hydroxybutyric acid, 50
Gender Dysphoria, 83, 85, 127
Generalized Anxiety Disorder (GAD),
  36, 37, 64
genito-pelvic pain/penetration
  disorder, 83, 84, 85
Geodon, 107
Gestalt Psychotherapy, 98
glue sniffing, 50
grief, 14
Group Therapy, 99
group/family/couples therapy, 95

Hair-Pulling Disorder, 40
Haldol, 107
hallucinogens, 49
haloperidol, 26, 27, 32, 107, 108, 125
Hamilton Depression Scale, 105
heroin, 48
HIPAA, 5
histamine H2 antagonists, 71
Histrionic Personality Disorder, 88
hoarding disorder, 40
humanistic therapy, 95
Huntington's chorea, 72
hydroxyzine, 42, 56, 112
hypercalcemia, 73
hypercarotenemia, 61
Hypersexual Disorder, 50
Hypersomnolence Disorder, 54
hyperthyroidism, 70
hypochondriasis, 64
hyponatremia, 73
hypothyroidism, 70
hysteria, 92
hysterical conversion, 92

id, 93
Illness Anxiety Disorder, 64
iloperidone, 25, 107, 108
imipramine, 100, 120

inhalant drugs, 50
Insomnia Disorder, 52
insulinomas, 38
Intellectual Disability, 80
Internet Use Disorder, 50
interpersonal psychoanalysis, 94
Interpersonal Psychotherapy, 18, 19, 99
Invega, 107
isocarboxazine, 105

Kayser-Fleischer rings, 124
Klonopin, 41

Lamictal, 110
lamotrigine, 31, 32, 110, 111
Latuda, 107
lead intoxication, 69
Levitra, 101
levomilnacipran, 103
Lewy Body Dementia, 34
Lexapro, 18, 102
Librium, 112
lithium, 30, 109, 122
loose associations, 8, 24, 126
lorazepam, 27, 32, 41, 47, 112
LOW FOOD, 57
loxapine, 26
Lunesta, 112
lurasidone, 25, 31, 32, 107, 108, 109

mania, 22
major depressive disorder, 19
Major Neurocognitive Disorder, 33
male hypoactive sexual desire
  disorder, 83, 84
malingering, 64, 66
manganese intoxication, 69
MAO inhibitor, 18, 20, 105
marijuana, 49
Marplan, 105
MED'CL, 69
melatonin, 56
Mellaril, 107
Mental Retardation, 80
mental status exam, 7

Mentalization-Based Therapy, 91, 95
meperidine, 48
meprobamate, 112
mercury poisoning, 69
metal poisoning, 69
methadone, 51
methylphenidate, 82
Mindfulness-Based Cognitive
    Therapy, 98
Mindfulness-Based Stress Reduction, 98
mirtazapine, 28, 19, 56, 103
modafinil, 106
monoamine oxidase inhibitors
    (MAOIs), 20, 100
mood stabilizers, 109
mood, 7
morphine, 48
Motivational Interviewing, 99
multiple personality disorder, 41
Munchausen Syndrome, 66

naltrexone, 47, 51, 113
Narcissistic Personality Disorder, 90,
    91
narcolepsy, 54
narcotics, 48
Nardil, 105
Navane, 107
nefazodone, 104
negative symptoms, 23
neologisms, 8
Neurocognitive Disorder with Lewy
    Bodies, 119
Neurontin, 111
nicotine, 50
night terrors, 77
Nightmare Disorder, 55
Norpramin, 100
nortriptyline, 104

obesity, 60
obsessions, 39
obsessive-compulsive disorder, 39
Obstructive Sleep Apnea Hypopnea, 54
OCPD, 39

oculogyric crisis, 109
odansetron, 113
olanzapine, 25, 26, 27, 31, 32, 107-111
olanzapine/fluoxetine, 109
operant conditioning, 96
opioids, 48
Oppositional Defiant Disorder (ODD),
    77
Other Specified Bipolar Disorder, 30
oxazepam, 47, 112
oxcarbazepine, 111
oxycodone, 48

pain in depression, 63
paint sniffing, 50
paliperidone, 27, 107, 108
panic disorder, 36, 37
paranoid (delusional) disorder, 25
paraphilic disorders, 83, 86
parasomnias, 55, 77
Parnate, 105
paroxetine, 18, 119, 43, 106, 101, 102,
    103, 112
pavor nocturnus, 77
Paxil, 18, 100
PCP, 50
pedophilia, 86
pedophilic disorder, 86
pellagra, 73
perphenazine, 26, 107, 108
perseveration, 8, 33
*Persistent Depressive Disorder
    (Dysthymia)*, 13
Person-Centered Psychotherapy, 98
personality disorders, 87
phenelzine, 20, 105
pheochromocytoma, 38, 72
phobias, 36, 37
pica, 61
polycystic ovary syndrome, 111
post-traumatic stress disorder (PTSD),
    40
prazosin, 43
premature (early) ejaculation, 83, 84, 85
primary anxiety, 36

Pristiq, 18, 103
Prolixin, 107
prolonged exposure therapy (PE), 42
propranolol and depression, 71
propranolol for anxiety, 42
Provigil, 106
Prozac, 18, 62, 100
pseudodementia, 14, 119
pseudoparkinsonism, 109
psychiatric evaluation, 6
psychodynamic model, 3
Psychodynamic Psychotherapy, 95
psychomotor retardation, 12
psychoses, 21
psychosis in children, 76
psychotherapy, 92
*Psychotic Disorder Due to Another
    Medical Condition*, 25
PTSD Dissociative Subtype, 41
PTSD, 40

quetiapine, 25, 31, 32, 107, 108, 109,
    110
Quick Inventory of Depressive
    Symptoms, 106

ramelteon, 56, 113
ranitidine, 71
Rapid Eye Movement Sleep Behavior
    Disorder, 55
relational psychoanalysis, 94
REM sleep, 52
Remeron, 18, 104
Restless Legs Syndrome, 55
Rett's Syndrome, 76
Revia, 113
Risperdal, 107
risperidone, 25, 26, 27, 107, 108, 110,
    124
Ritalin, 82
Rozerem, 113

sadomasochism, 86
Saphris, 107
Schema Therapy, 91

schizoaffective disorder, 25
Schizoid Personality Disorder, 87
Schizotypal Personality Disorder, 88
Schizophreniform Disorder, 24
schizophrenia, 21, 22, 23
second-generation antipsychotics
    (SGA), 26, 107, 108
sedative-hypnotics, 112
sedatives, 49
selective mutism, 79
Separation Anxiety Disorder, 79
Serax, 112
Seroquel, 107
serotonin selective reuptake inhibitors
    (SSRIs), 42
serotonin syndrome, 106
sertraline, 18, 19, 20, 43, 101, 102,
    106, 112, 117
Serzone, 104
sexual dysfunctions, 83
sexual masochism disorder, 86
sexual sadism disorder, 86
sildenafil, 101
Sinequan, 100
sleep apnea, 54
sleep talking, 77
sleep terrors, 55
Sleep-Related Hypoventilation, 54
sleepless patient, 52
sleepwalking, 55
SNRIs, 103
social anxiety disorder, 36, 37
Social Communication Disorder, 76
social phobia, 36, 37
Somatic Delusional Disorder, 25
somatic symptom disorder, 64
somnambulism, 55, 77
somniloquy, 77
Spice/K2, 50
splitting, 93
SSRIs, 42, 100
St. John's Wort, 106
Stelazine, 107
Stevens-Johnson syndrome, 111
stimulants, 49

Strattera, 82
substance use disorders, 44
Substance-induced Psychotic Disorder, 25
Substance/Medication Induced Depressive Disorder, 13
Substance/Medication-Induced Bipolar Disorder, 30
substance/medication-induced sexual dysfunction, 84
SUICIDAL, 16
suicide, 11, 15
superego, 93
Symbyax, 110
systematic desensitization, 96

tadalafil, 101
tangential thought, 8
tardive dyskinesia, 109, 119
TCAs, 18
temazepam, 47, 55
temporal lobe epilepsy, 38
thiamine deficiency in alcoholism, 46
thioridazine, 107
thiothixene, 107, 108
Thorazine, 107
thought blocking, 8
tic disorder, 80
timolol, 71
TMS, 19
Tofranil, 100
Topamax, 112, 113
topiramate, 112, 113
Tourette's syndrome, 80
transcranial magnetic stimulation, 19, 114
Transference Focused Psychotherapy, 91, 95
transference, 2, 94
transvestic disorder, 86
transvestism, 86
Tranxene, 112
tranylcypromine, 20, 105
trazodone, 56, 104
treatment modalities, 92

triazolam, 56, 113
trichotillomania, 40
tricyclic antidepressants (TCAs), 18, 100
trifluoperazine, 26, 107, 108
Trilafon, 107
Trileptal, 111
Trintellix, 101

undoing, 93
unipolar depression, 11
Unspecified Bipolar Disorder, 30
Unspecified Delusional Disorder, 25
Unspecified Depressive Disorder, 13

VACUUM, 78
Valium, 41
valproate, 31
valproic acid, 31
vardenafil, 101
Vascular Dementia, 34
vegetative signs of depression, 13
venlafaxine, 10, 18, 19, 103, 106, 112
Viagra, 101
Viibryd, 101
vilazodone, 101
vitamin B12 deficiency, 73
vortioxetine, 101, 104
voyeuristic disorder, 86

waxy flexibility, 24
Wellbutrin, 18
Wernicke-Korsakoff syndrome, 46
Wilson's disease, 65, 72, 124
word salad, 8

Xanax, 41, 112, 124

zaleplon, 112
ziprasidone, 25, 27, 107, 108, 109
Zofran, 113
Zoloft, 18, 102
zolpidem, 55, 112
Zonegran, 112
zonesimide, 112
Zyprexa, 107, 110